In Vitro Fertilization

The A.R.T. of Making Babies

Third Edition

Geoffrey Sher, M.D.
Virginia Marriage Davis, R.N., M.N.
Jean Stoess, M.A.

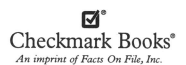

Checkmark Books®

An imprint of Facts On File, Inc.

In Vitro Fertilization: The A.R.T. of Making Babies, Third Edition

Checkmark Books
An imprint of Infobase Publishing
132 West 31st Street
New York NY 10001

ISBN-10: 0-8160-6053-3
ISBN-13: 978-0-8160-6053-5

Library of Congress Cataloging-in-Publication Data
Sher, Geoffrey, 1943–
    In vitro fertilization : the a.r.t. of making babies / Geoffrey Sher, Virginia Marriage Davis, Jean Stoess.—3rd ed.
        p. cm.
    Includes bibliographical references and index.
    ISBN 0-8160-6047-9 (hc : alk. paper)—ISBN 0-8160-6053-3 (pb : alk. paper)
    1. Fertilization in vitro, Human—Popular works. 2. Human reproductive technology—Popular works. I. Davis, Virginia Marriage. II. Stoess, Jean. III. Title.
    RG135.S543 2004
    618.1'78059—dc22   2004008105

Checkmark Books are available at special discounts when purchased in bulk quantities for businesses, associations, institutions, or sales promotions. Please call our Special Sales Department in New York at (212) 967-8800 or (800) 322-8755.

You can find Facts On File on the World Wide Web at
http://www.factsonfile.com

Text design adapted by James Scotto-Lavino
Cover design by Nora Wertz
Illustrations by Marc Greene and Dale Williams

Printed in the United States of America

MP FOF 10 9 8 7 6 5 4

This book is printed on acid-free paper.

*This book is dedicated to the memory of
Virginia Marriage Davis, R.N., M.N.,
one of the co-authors of previous editions of the book,
who died recently of breast cancer.*

*Virginia was instrumental in developing and refining the
IVF program at the Northern Nevada Fertility Center in Reno, NV,
upon which the material in this book was originally based.
As nurse-coordinator of the program, Virginia was the ultimate
patient advocate. Her unfailing efforts to make the IVF experience
as positive as possible for the infertile couple, whether or not they
had a baby, and the understanding and warmth with which she
interacted with them are reflected in many of the quotes throughout
this book, such as her comments about the emotional toll that
induction of ovulation imposes on women and the importance of
using visualization for relaxation during embryo transfer,
as well as the quote about the positive aspects of the process by a
woman who underwent IVF but was unable to conceive.*

*Virginia Marriage Davis was a medical practice consultant,
family nurse practitioner, and lecturer who spoke
internationally about infertility and women's reproductive rights.
She is survived by her husband and two children.*

CONTENTS

FOREWORD

by Nancy Hemenway

Designer egg auctions, cloning, and "test-tube babies" are all "hot topics" used by the media to fuel the controversial fires surrounding infertility treatment options. More than 5 million couples are faced with the prospect of navigating and filtering a colossal maze of information and misinformation in order to successfully build their families. This winding road to family can be extremely lonely, physically demanding, and emotionally draining. Dr. Geoffrey Sher is a cool oasis and breath of fresh air for couples embarking on this exhausting journey.

Dr. Geoffrey Sher, executive medical director of Sher Institutes for Reproductive Medicine, practicing in Las Vegas, Nevada, and New York, New York, is one of a kind. He is entrepreneurial, energetic, passionate, and compassionate in his approach to both the science and medical aspects of reproductive medicine. Dr. Sher's book *In Vitro Fertilization, the A.R.T of Making Babies,* with coauthors Virginia Marriage Davis, R.N., M.N., and Jean Stoess, M.A., is a beacon and road map for those plotting their treatment course.

The A.R.T. of Making Babies empowers the individual with reliable information, in down-to-earth language. Sher's forward-thinking and frank dialogue tackles difficult and controversial topics with honesty and integrity. Together the authors further the idea that working in tandem with one's physician to build a family should be the rule—not the exception.

Over the last 15 years, I have been an advocate, educator, a patient, a consumer, and, finally, after years of navigating the infertility labyrinth, a parent twice blessed. I am a survivor of many infertility battles and the cofounder and executive director of the InterNational Council on

Infertility Information Dissemination, Inc. (INCIID—pronounced "inside"), the world's largest infertility advocacy organization. I've worked alongside some of the leading names in the field of reproductive medicine. Yet there is none I am more honored to call friend and colleague than Geoffrey Sher, M.D.; a man of many talents, who has a clear vision for the future.

FOREWORD
by Pamela Madsen

Innovative, insightful, skillful and compassionate. It is this rare combination that distinguishes Dr. Geoffrey Sher and has earned him the respect of peers and patients alike. His creativity in the battle against infertility goes beyond the science and practice of assisted reproduction. It encompasses patient education and access to care. Indeed, the Sher Institutes for Reproductive Medicine pioneered risk-sharing, a once-controversial financing arrangement that makes assisted reproductive technology (ART) treatments more affordable.

As executive director and founder of the American Infertility Association (AIA), the largest infertility patient organization in the United States, I've had the pleasure of working with Dr. Sher. His dedication to patient welfare is unquestionable.

The ART of Making Babies, coauthored with Virginia Marriage Davis, R.N., M.N., and Jean Stoess, M.A., is true to Dr. Sher's convictions. With its clear language and conversational tone, the book reflects Dr. Sher's belief that communicating with patients enables them to become their own best advocates and partners in care.

The reliable and comprehensive information within these pages is invaluable to the thousands of people who find themselves confused, lost, and frightened by infertility. With honesty and empathy, the authors make even the most complex technical medical material accessible and understandable. They tackle the thorny issues of money, insurance, emotion, and ethics with a generosity of spirit that not only raises the tough questions but provides some tools for dealing with them as well.

As a veteran of the infertility wars, I can say without hesitation that this book is a resource treasure. Read it and take heart.

PREFACE

Innovators are rarely received with joy, and established authorities launch into condemnation of newer truths; for at every crossroad to the future are a thousand self-appointed guardians of the past.

—Betty MacQuitty, *Victory Over Pain: Morton's Discovery of Anesthesia*

In vitro fertilization (IVF) has come a long way since 1978, when Louise Brown, christened "the world's first test-tube baby" by the press, was born in England. The first in vitro fertilization program in the United States was introduced at the Eastern Virginia Medical School at Norfolk in the late 1970s. Now, about 400 clinics throughout the United States offer IVF, with varying degrees of reported success.

In vitro fertilization literally means "fertilization in glass." Traditionally known as in vitro fertilization and embryo transfer (IVF/ET), the procedure is more commonly referred to simply as in vitro fertilization, or IVF. (The term IVF will be used throughout this book instead of the more cumbersome IVF/ET.)

IVF is composed of several basic steps. First, the woman is given fertility drugs that stimulate her ovaries to produce as many mature eggs as possible. Then, when the ovaries have been properly stimulated, the eggs are retrieved by suction through a needle inserted into her ovaries. The harvested eggs are then fertilized in a petri dish in the laboratory with her partner's or a donor's sperm. Several days later, the fertilized egg(s)—now known as embryo(s)—are transferred by a thin catheter through the woman's vagina into her uterus, where it is hoped they will grow into one or more healthy babies.

It is essential that the infertile couple and their physician identify the cause of the infertility in order to determine the most appropriate form of treatment. This does not mean that IVF should be regarded as a treatment of last resort. It may well be that IVF offers the best hope for a healthy pregnancy. At most reputable IVF centers, the chance of a woman becoming pregnant with IVF is much greater than that of a fertile woman conceiving (without treatment) in any given month of trying. Nevertheless, the couple should understand that IVF is not everything to everyone and that some women never get pregnant through IVF, no matter how many times they try.

Many infertile couples who have experienced repeated disappointments over the years in their attempts to conceive have become desperate. Most have previously tried a variety of unsuccessful procedures: fertility drugs for the woman and/or man, medications to treat various hormonal problems, nonsurgical alternatives such as artificial insemination, and pelvic surgery to repair anatomical defects. All these couples look to IVF as a promising procedure that might help them conceive after all of their other attempts have failed.

Yet, of the more than 2.5 million couples in the United States for whom IVF offers the best option for pregnancy, less than 250,000 undergo the procedure annually. Clearly, eligible infertile couples in the United States are not even coming close to tapping into the potential of IVF. Why is this so?

One reason is that some people still consider IVF to be experimental. However, the evidence proves otherwise—about 300,000 IVF babies have already been born in the United States. Yet the public, in company with many members of the medical profession, still knows relatively little about IVF beyond the way it is characterized by the media.

People get a distorted idea about IVF when they turn on the television and see a slide of a test tube with a baby inside. By no means either a test tube or a baby are involved at that point. There are just a momentary couple of days when fertilization takes place outside the body, and then the embryo(s) is placed in the woman's uterus and begins to grow there. The phrase *test-tube baby* is a convenient handle for the media, but it misleadingly implies that the whole process occurs outside the body, which is not true.

Unfortunately, consumers find it difficult to get much in-depth information about this exciting procedure. (The term *consumers* is used here to mean both infertile couples and physicians who refer their patients to a particular program.) Currently, no credible source provides prospectively audited, verifiable information about success rates obtained from IVF programs in the United States. As a result, people trying to learn about IVF often feel as though they are stumbling in the dark.

Several national organizations, including the Society for Assisted Reproductive Technology (SART), an affiliated society of the American Society for Reproductive Medicine (ASRM), and a number of support groups for infertile couples provide limited information about IVF and related procedures. SART was formed in 1988 under the umbrella of the ASRM, which is primarily made up of physicians but also includes laboratory personnel, psychologists, nurses, and other paramedical personnel interested in infertility.

SART provides a list of IVF programs in the United States, but it does not recommend or endorse any specific programs. Instead, SART encourages consumers to contact IVF programs individually for more information. (Society for Assisted Reproductive Technology, 1209 Montgomery Highway, Birmingham, AL 35216; telephone: (205) 978-5000; fax: (205) 978-5015; Web site: http://www.sart.org.)

Aside from the problem of insufficient information, another obstacle to widespread acceptance of IVF is its high cost. IVF is relatively expensive—$7,000 to $15,000 per procedure, depending on the program.

Many couples pass up IVF because of the financial burden, although it may be the most appropriate treatment for them. They simply can't afford it. Some states have passed laws requiring insurance companies to reimburse in total for IVF, and several others are considering similar legislation. Nevertheless, we must inform consumers that a new form of payment for IVF services known as Outcome Based Reimbursement (OBR) promises to make IVF services more affordable. More than 70 IVF programs in the United States currently offer OBR in one form or another, and the number is growing. (See chapter 16 for a discussion about OBR and the need for insurance reimbursement for IVF.)

Yet we must also warn consumers that the outlook on IVF-related issues is not likely to improve for some time. IVF will remain an expensive procedure. But by researching the IVF situation for themselves, couples will be able to answer these fundamental questions: (1) Are we eligible for IVF? and (2) How do we select the program that will give us the best results?

This book is designed to help answer these critical questions. It describes IVF and some other assisted reproductive technology (ART) procedures; outlines a variety of emotional, physical, financial, and moral/religious issues; and highlights points that should be considered when deciding whether IVF or another high-tech procedure is indeed the most appropriate option. We do not offer any judgments relating to ethics, religion, or morality. These kinds of decisions are private matters that must be resolved by each couple in their own way. We do not intend to imply that our approach is the only acceptable way and/or should be rigidly followed. Our function is to recommend, to inform, to educate, and to serve—but never to dictate.

We are particularly cognizant of the fact that many women who do conceive following IVF may have pregnancies that are at risk. Going from infertility to family can be extremely traumatic from an emotional, psychological, and physical point of view. One of the ways we prepare couples is by providing them with as much information about infertility, as well as IVF and related procedures, as they need. We believe that being as knowledgeable as possible helps them cope with the roller-coaster experience they will undergo.

Accordingly, we will be glad to provide the readers of this book any information they might request about infertility. To request this material, call (800) 780-7437 or obtain additional information by accessing the Sher Institutes for Reproductive Medicine (SIRM) Web site at www.haveababy.com. *In Vitro Fertilization: The A.R.T. of Making Babies* may also be purchased via the Internet at http://www.factsonfile.com or www.amazon.com.

Finally, we wrote this book to help consumers develop and maintain realistic expectations about IVF. Realistic expectations revolve around the best and the worst possible scenarios; but all infertile couples should prepare themselves for the worst, just in case. However, by planning an effective strategy, asking the right questions, and evaluating the answers properly, candidates can determine whether they are eligible for IVF and can find the most appropriate program. As a 35-year-old new mother told us, doing that homework does pay off:

I must have spent at least three hours talking with my own physician, trying to find out where to go for IVF. It was so frustrating not being able to find anyone who could give me any real answers. Several times I was tempted to go to the IVF clinic nearest us just because it was so convenient. But, thank God, I did my homework as thoroughly as I knew how. I must have called up fifteen different programs. I asked a lot of questions about success rates and what it was like to go through their programs, and then I had to sort everything out. I finally found a great program—and now we have a beautiful little girl who is the joy of our lives. I can hardly remember what life had been like without her. It was worth all that effort.

—Geoffrey Sher, M.D.

UNITS OF MEASUREMENT

The following abbreviations for units of measurement are used in this book.

cc   cubic centimeter
cm   centimeter
mcg   microgram
mg   milligram
miu   milli-international unit
ml   milliliter
mm   millimeter
ng   nanogram
pg   picogram

1

THE GROWING DILEMMA OF INFERTILITY

It is estimated that there are about 45 million couples of childbearing age living together in the United States today. Approximately 5 million of these couples are infertile.

This estimate is based on a series of nationwide surveys of cohabiting married couples in which the women were between 15 and 44 years of age. It was found that one out of every 12 couples, or 8 percent, were involuntarily infertile.

Infertility can be defined as the inability to conceive after one full year of normal, regular heterosexual intercourse without the use of any contraception. The odds that a woman will get pregnant without medical assistance when she has failed to do so after a year or two of unprotected intercourse are extremely low.

Only couples who have experienced the problem of infertility can truly understand its devastating emotional and physical impacts. As one woman who had been trying unsuccessfully to become pregnant for many years explained:

It has been two years since I learned the reason I wasn't getting pregnant was because my fallopian tubes were blocked. It is incredible to think that I have had more physical assault on my body in the last two years than in the rest of my thirty years combined. I underwent it voluntarily, too, because I wanted to correct the problem and have a child. Yet all the surgeries, the tests, and the medications seemed relatively minor compared to the emotional burden I put on myself.

After my first surgery, when my physician said it was okay to try to become pregnant, I don't think there was ever a day, or perhaps even an hour, that I didn't think about conceiving. It was always there—when I would see a child in the grocery store. When my friends would gripe about their kids. When I was on day 1, or day 14, and every other day of my menstrual cycle. Whenever my husband and I made love. Was I ever going to get pregnant? I had conflicting fantasies of what I would be like as a 60-year-old woman who had never had children. I could never get it out of my mind.

One study of infertile couples illustrates the pervasive impact of infertility. When asked what they considered to be the primary problem in their lives, almost 80 percent of the couples replied that it was their inability to conceive. Most of the remaining 20 percent ranked infertility as their second most perplexing problem, after financial difficulties. The remaining fraction of respondents rated infertility a close third after financial problems and marital strife.

A newly pregnant woman, who had just completed her second IVF treatment cycle, summed up the emotional impact of infertility in this way:

You really can't understand what it's like to be infertile unless you are infertile yourself and have experienced what we've gone through. You can sympathize, but you can't empathize with us.

The traditional options available to infertile couples who want a baby have included counseling, surgery to repair anatomical damage, the use of fertility drugs to enhance ovulation and sperm function, and insemination of the woman with her partner's or a donor's sperm. Most authorities would agree that these methods are effective for approximately 50 percent of all infertile couples. For the about 2.5 million infertile couples in the United States, IVF is the only recourse; yet fewer than 250,000 procedures are being performed annually.

WHY THE NUMBER OF INFERTILE COUPLES IN THE UNITED STATES IS INCREASING EVERY YEAR
___

According to the National Center for Health Statistics, the rate of involuntary infertility has remained constant at about 8.5 percent since 1965. This is an increase over the figures for the early 1950s through 1964, when it was thought that approximately 7–8 percent of all couples were unable to conceive. Although the rate of infertility has not changed since the mid-1960s, the number of infertile couples has increased every year in step with population growth. The following factors contribute to this trend.

Venereal Diseases Are Epidemic in the United States

Once considered largely under control because of the discovery and availability of proper medication, venereal diseases that damage the reproductive system are on the rise again. One of the major causes of this is the increased availability of effective birth control methods, which has undoubtedly contributed to a more open approach toward sexual activity. Consequently, both men and women often have relatively large numbers of sexual partners. The unfortunate result has been a significant increase in sexually transmitted diseases.

Venereal diseases such as gonorrhea are rampant in the United States. Gonorrhea lodges in the woman's fallopian tubes and often results in a severe illness. Unfortunately, in many cases gonorrhea causes so little physical discomfort that women frequently do not bother to seek treatment. But even a minor gonorrheal infection can damage the fallopian tubes, and many women find out they have had gonorrhea only when they investigate the cause of their infertility. In contrast, gonorrhea in men almost always produces sudden, painful symptoms that usually prompt an immediate visit to the doctor. For this reason, men are less likely to be infertile due to gonorrhea than are women.

The cure of sexually transmitted diseases is complicated by the emergence of new strains of gonorrhea and other venereal diseases that resist traditional treatment. These bacteria can be combated only by new and expensive antibiotics that often are not readily available.

Chlamydia, another infection that damages and blocks the fallopian tubes, is even more common today than gonorrhea. Chlamydia is relatively difficult to diagnose and culture, and it responds well only to specific antibiotics. Past infection is diagnosed through a specific staining procedure of cervical secretions or by blood testing for anti-chlamydia antibodies. The symptoms of chlamydia are very similar to those of gonorrhea.

Syphilis, too, is again becoming widespread in the United States. Syphilis is easily cured in its early stages. In later stages its spread can be halted, but its effects cannot be reversed.

(See "Pelvic Inflammatory Diseases" in chapter 9 for a discussion of the effect of sexually transmitted diseases on infertility.)

Medications and "Recreational Drugs" Are Taking Their Toll

Alcohol, nicotine, marijuana, cocaine, and other psychotropic drugs can significantly reduce both male and female fertility because they are capable of altering the genetic material of eggs and sperm. However, these substances can potentially have a far more severe and long-lasting effect on a woman than on a man. Because a woman is born with her lifetime quota of eggs already inside her ovaries, unwise use of medications and drugs can damage all the eggs her body will ever produce (see chapter 8). In contrast, a man generates a completely new supply of sperm approximately every three months, so damaged sperm are replaced in a short time.

The Biological Clock Keeps on Ticking

Many women today choose to delay having a family in order to establish their careers, to be sure they and their partner can afford children because they married relatively late, or because they want to have a child with a new partner. However, there is a price to pay for having children later on. For example, some disorders that produce infertility tend to appear during the second half of a woman's reproductive life span. Thus, a woman who decides to have children after 35 might find she is infertile because of hormonal problems, a pelvic disease such as endometriosis, or the development of benign fibroid tumors of the uterus. In addition, the ability to ovulate healthy eggs and concurrently generate a hormonal environment that can adequately support a pregnancy becomes increasingly compromised as a woman gets older (see chapter 8). Many women who plan to become pregnant later in their reproductive lives find themselves unable to do so.

Although the infertility rate has not increased, the aggregate number of couples whose last option for pregnancy is IVF is skyrocketing. Recent advances in the evolution of high-tech methods to evaluate and treat infertility offer the hope of pregnancy to couples who previously would have had no hope. To date, about 300,000 very special miracles have been granted the gift of life through assisted reproductive technology (ART) in the United States.

2

THE ANATOMY AND PHYSIOLOGY OF REPRODUCTION

In vitro fertilization can be viewed as an extension of the normal human reproductive process. It merely bypasses many of the anatomical or physiological causes of infertility by substituting IVF techniques for some of the processes that occur naturally in the body. In order to understand both natural conception and IVF, therefore, one must first be familiar with human reproductive anatomy and the process of reproduction.

THE FEMALE REPRODUCTIVE TRACT

The female reproductive tract consists of the vulva, vagina, cervix, uterus, fallopian tubes, and ovaries. The external portion of the female reproductive tract (see figure 2-1) is known as the *vulva.* The vulva includes the inner and outer lips, or *labia.* The hair-covered outer labia are called the *labia majora* (major lips). The *labia minora,* small inner lips partially hidden by the labia majora, are remnants of tissue whose embryologic counterpart in the male develops into the scrotum.

The *clitoris,* a small organ at the junction of the labia minora in the front of the vulva, is the embryologic counterpart of the male penis. The clitoris undergoes erection during erotic stimulation and plays an important role in orgasm.

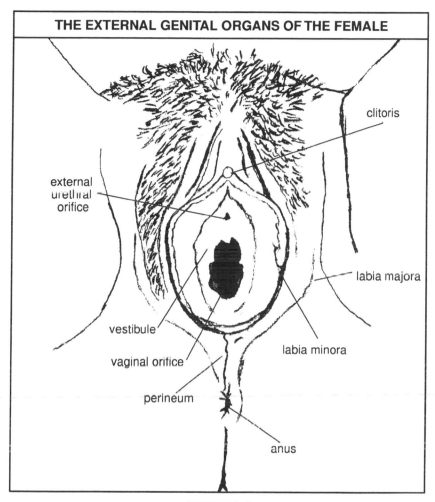

THE EXTERNAL GENITAL ORGANS OF THE FEMALE

clitoris

external
urethral
orifice

labia majora

vestibule

labia minora

vaginal orifice

perineum

anus

FIGURE 2-1

The area between the labia minora and the anus is called the *perineum.* It is formed by the outer portion of the fibromuscular wall and skin that separate the *anus* and *rectum* from the vagina and vulva.

The *vagina,* a narrow passage about 3½–4 inches long and about 1 inch wide, spans the area between the vulva and the cervix. It opens outward through the cleft between the labia minora, or *vestibule.* The

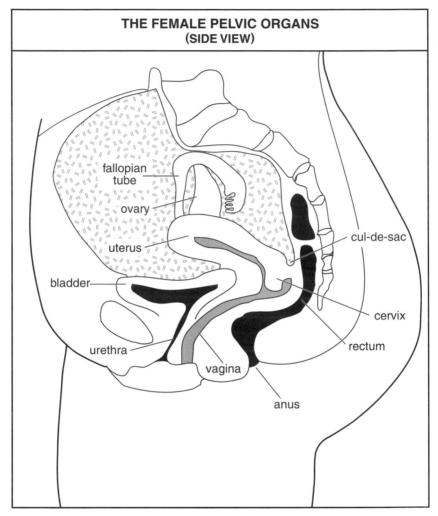

THE FEMALE PELVIC ORGANS (SIDE VIEW)

FIGURE 2-2

vagina's elastic tissue, muscle, and skin have enormous ability to stretch so as to accommodate the penis during the sex act and the passage of a baby at birth. The vagina is actually a potential space; it is a real space only when the penis enters it or during childbirth. At other times, the vaginal walls are collapsed against one another; a cross section of a relaxed vagina would resemble the letter H. In front of the vagina lie the

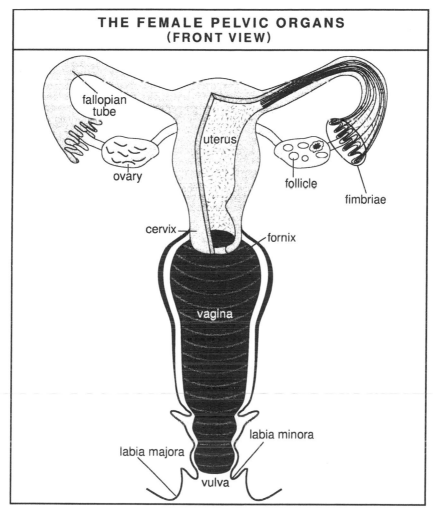

THE FEMALE PELVIC ORGANS
(FRONT VIEW)

fallopian
tube

uterus

ovary

follicle

fimbriae

cervix

fornix

vagina

labia minora

labia majora

vulva

FIGURE 2-3

bladder and the *urethra* (outlet from the bladder), and at the back is the rectum (see figure 2-2).

The cervix, which is the lowermost part of the uterus, protrudes like a bottleneck into the upper vagina. As figure 2-3 illustrates, a *fornix,* or deep recess, is created around the area where the cervix extends into the vagina. The area of the abdominal cavity behind the uterus is known as the *cul-de-sac.* The cervix opens into the uterus through a narrow canal, the lining of which contains glands that produce cervical mucus (the important role that cervical mucus plays in the reproductive process will be explained later in this chapter). The cervix is particularly vulnerable to infections and other diseases, such as cancer.

The *uterus,* which consists of strong muscle fibers, is able to stretch and grow from its normal size (when it resembles a pear) to accommodate a full-term pregnancy. The valvelike transition between the cervix and the uterine cavity enables a baby to grow within the uterus without prematurely dilating the cervix and thereby endangering the pregnancy through miscarriage or premature birth. The lining of the uterus, which nurtures and supports the developing embryo, is known as the *endometrium.*

The *fallopian tubes* are two narrow 4-inch-long structures that lead from either side of the uterus to the ovaries. At the end of the fallopian tubes are finger-like protrusions known as *fimbriae.*

The *ovaries* are two almond-sized structures attached to each side of the pelvis adjacent to the fimbriae. The ovaries both release eggs and discharge certain hormones into the bloodstream. The process of releasing the egg or eggs is called *ovulation.* Eggs are also known as *ova* or *oocytes.*

About the size of a grain of sand, eggs are the largest cells in the human body. A woman develops all the eggs she will ever have at the fetal age of 12 weeks. Although a female baby starts off with about 7 million eggs when she is inside her mother's womb, her ovaries contain only about 700,000 eggs by the time she reaches puberty. A woman uses about 300,000 of these eggs during the approximately 400 ovulations that occur during her reproductive life span.

Each month, the ovaries select a number of the woman's eggs for maturation. Eggs mature in blister-like structures, or *follicles,* that project from the surface of the ovaries. At ovulation, the egg is not simply expelled into the abdominal cavity. Instead, the fimbriae at the ends of the fallopian tubes gently vacuum the surface of the ovaries to retrieve the egg and direct it through the fallopian tubes for possible fertilization.

The human egg (see figure 2-4) is similar in structure to the eggs of many other species, including the chicken. In the center of the human

A HUMAN EGG

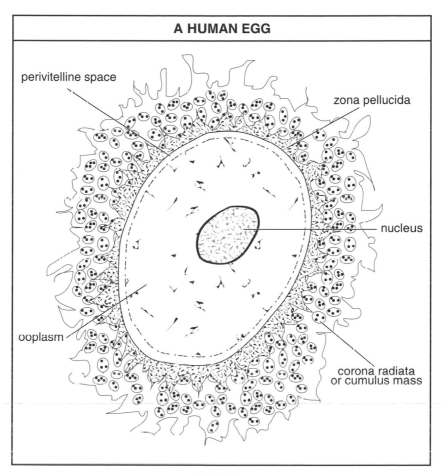

FIGURE 2-4

egg is the *nucleus,* which bears the chromosomes. The surrounding *ooplasm* contains *micro-organelles,* which are cellular factories that produce energy for the egg. The ooplasm also contains nurturing material that supports the embryo during its early stages after fertilization, thus enabling it to grow before becoming attached to an external source of nourishment (the endometrium). Surrounding the ooplasm and nuclear material is the *perivitelline membrane,* which separates the internal matter from the *zona pellucida.* The zona pellucida is analogous to the shell of a chicken egg, and the perivitelline membrane corresponds to the membrane inside the eggshell. The human egg, unlike the chicken egg, also contains a group of cells known as the *cumulus granulosa*, which are arranged in a starburst effect around the outside of the zona pellucida. (The critical role each of these structures plays in the fertilization process is explained later in this chapter under "How Fertilization Occurs.")

THE MALE REPRODUCTIVE TRACT

The male sex organs (see figure 2-5) comprise the *penis* and two *testicles*, or *testes*, which are located in a sac called the *scrotum*. The testicles (male counterparts of the woman's ovaries) produce *spermatozoa*, or *sperm* (the male equivalent of the woman's eggs).

In contrast to the woman, who is born with a lifetime quota of eggs, the man's testicles generate a new complement of sperm approximately every 100 days. The sperm begin to mature in the testicles and continue to develop as they travel through a long, thin, coiled tubular system in the scrotum called the *epididymis*. The epididymis is connected to a straight, thicker tube called the *vas deferens*. Just before the vas deferens enters the penis it joins the *urethra*, which originates in the bladder and allows the passage of urine from the bladder through the penis. Sperm are transported through this system by muscular contractions known as *peristalsis*.

Several glands, including the *seminal vesicles* and the *prostate gland*, are located along this tract. They release a large amount of milky secretions that nurture and promote the survival of the sperm. The combination of sperm and milky fluid that is ejaculated during erotic experiences is known as *semen*. Semen and urine are not discharged simultaneously through the urethra. Urine is prevented from mixing with semen in the urethra because the bladder-urethra opening constricts during ejaculation. Similarly, closure of the vas deferens–urethra juncture prevents passage of semen during urination. In certain cases, removal of a diseased prostate gland may compromise this separation effect and cause the man to ejaculate backward into the bladder rather than outward through the

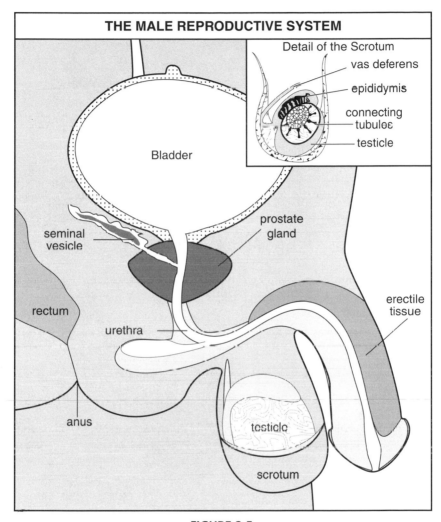

FIGURE 2-5

penis, which is known as *retrograde ejaculation*. This condition may cause infertility, but it can be treated by inseminating the woman with sperm separated from urine the man would pass immediately following orgasm.

Sperm (see figure 2-6), in contrast to eggs, are the smallest cells in the body. They resemble microscopic tadpoles. Each sperm consists of

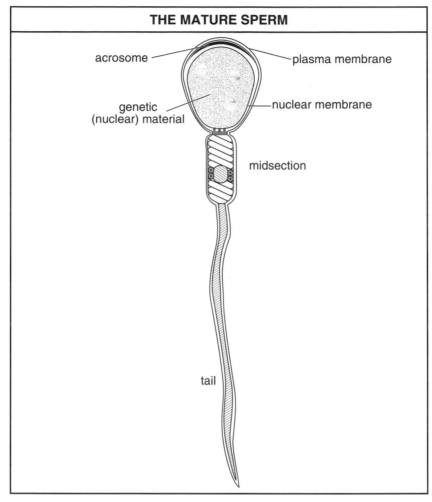

THE MATURE SPERM

acrosome — plasma membrane

genetic (nuclear) material — nuclear membrane

midsection

tail

FIGURE 2-6

a head, whose *nucleus* contains the genetic, or hereditary, material arrayed on chromosomes; a midsection that provides energy; and a tail that propels the sperm along the male reproductive system and through the woman's reproductive tract. The top of the head is covered by the *acrosome,* a protective structure containing enzymes that enable the sperm to penetrate the egg; and the surface of the acrosome is enveloped by the *plasma membrane.* (The function of the acrosome and plasma membrane will be explained under "How Fertilization Occurs" later in this chapter.)

Eggs and sperm are called *gametes* until fertilization. A fertilized egg is called a *zygote* until it begins to divide; from initial cell division through the first eight weeks of gestation it is known as an *embryo,* and from the ninth week of gestation until delivery it is called a *fetus.*

HOW THE GENETIC BLUEPRINT IS DRAWN

Each cell in a human being (except for the gametes) contain 46 chromosomes, which are bound together into 23 pairs. Chromosomes contain hundreds of thousands of genes, each of which transmits the hereditary messages of the man or woman.

If a sperm containing 46 chromosomes were to fertilize an egg that also contained 46 chromosomes, it is obvious that the two gametes would produce a zygote containing double the proper number of chromosomes. Therefore, nature has created a method through which the number of chromosomes in both the sperm and egg is reduced by half. This reduction-division, which occurs immediately prior to and during fertilization, is referred to as *meiosis* (see figure 2-7).

As a result of this process, a newly fertilized zygote also contains 46 chromosomes. All that has been exchanged is the chromosomal material, including the genes. This simple-looking cell is actually quite complex, for within its boundaries lies the information for 100,000 chemical reactions: the blueprint for a new individual. The set of instructions carried on the chromosomes is complete, and a virtual explosion of embryonic development is imminent.

When the cells of the zygote begin to divide, and continue to divide over and over, they replicate the same number of chromosomes that occurred in the zygote. Thus, every new cell has 23 identical pairs of chromosomes (46 total chromosomes) in its own new image. Such division for the purpose of replicating cells identically is called *mitosis.* The growth and development of all tissues—with the exception, of course, of the gametes—is done by mitosis. Obviously, such a sensitive, intricate mechanism can and often does go wrong. Because this process

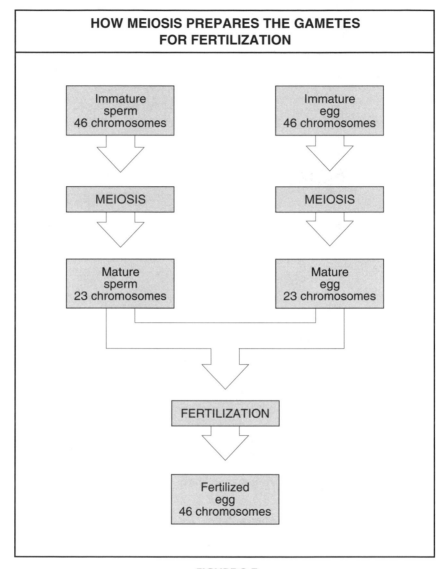

FIGURE 2-7

malfunctions so often, nature has devised a way of selecting out its mistakes and discarding them. (This will be discussed at the end of the chapter under "Miscarriage in Early Pregnancy.")

THE PROCESS OF FERTILIZATION

Fertilization is a complex process that must be accomplished within a strict time frame. Theoretically, a man is always fertile, but a woman's egg can only be fertilized within a specific 12- to 24-hour period shortly after ovulation. Therefore, there is a "window of opportunity" lasting only 24 to 48 hours each month when intercourse can be expected to result in fertilization. Timing is critical if the egg and sperm are to survive the journey through the woman's reproductive tract, unite, become fertilized, and result in the embryo implanting successfully into the uterine wall.

The man deposits between 100 million and 200 million sperm into the woman's vagina with each ejaculation of semen. During normal intercourse, or even after the woman has been artificially inseminated, much of the semen pools in the posterior fornix behind the protruding cervix. Because the cervix usually points partially backward into the posterior fornix, the cervix is usually immersed in the pool of ejaculated semen. This immersion helps direct the sperm through the cervix and into the reproductive tract.

The journey from the fornix to the fallopian tubes, which is about four inches, is hazardous and unbelievably taxing for the tiny sperm. For a cell the size of a sperm to travel this distance is equivalent to an adult human swimming the Pacific Ocean from Los Angeles to Tahiti. Only a small fraction of exceptionally strong, healthy sperm out of several million that were deposited in the fornix will survive that 24- to 48-hour journey. Many are killed by the hostile environment in the vagina or cervix, and others simply do not survive the long swim. Peristaltic contractions in the fallopian tubes help the remaining sperm reach the egg, and the same contractions propel the fertilized egg or embryo back through the fallopian tube to the uterus. (The fertilization process occurs near the middle of the fallopian tube—not in the uterus.) Amazingly, out of the millions of sperm ejaculated into the vagina, only a few hundred to a few thousand successfully complete the journey to the waiting egg in the fallopian tube.

An egg presents a large target for the tiny sperm: about $1/180$-inch as opposed to the sperm's $1/100,000$-inch diameter. This means that the egg is about 550 times as wide as the sperm. The difference in size between the two gametes is due to the massive amount of cytoplasm within the egg that will nourish the newly formed embryo. Sperm, in contrast, consist almost entirely of genetic material with very little cytoplasm. They are little more than bags of chromosomes propelled by a tail.

IVF improves the odds that sperm can find and fertilize an egg. This is because the distance sperm have to swim to find the egg in a petri dish is considerably shorter than the "long-distance route to Tahiti" found in nature. The egg still lies passively within the dish, as it would in the fallopian tube; but in the significantly reduced volume of the petri dish, the sperm are far more likely to find the egg than they would be if they had to negotiate the entire distance from the fornix.

How Fertilization Occurs

The process whereby sperm are prepared to fertilize an egg, which is known as *capacitation,* takes place in two stages. First, as a sperm passes through the woman's reproductive tract, its acrosome fuses with its plasma membrane, slowly releasing the enzymes within the acrosome. Then, with its acrosome now exposed, the sperm attacks the cumulus granulosa and the zona pellucida (the shell-like covering) of the egg. The heads of a number of sperm fuse with the zona pellucida, and one successful sperm penetrates the egg. The process whereby a sperm fuses with the zona, the second state of capacitation, is called the *acrosome reaction.* The sperm require from five to 10 hours of incubation in the fluids of the female reproductive tract to complete the acrosome reaction.

Capacitation takes place in the mucus secretions of the cervical canal, and continues in the uterus and fallopian tubes. It is believed that the passage of sperm through the cervical mucus around the time of ovulation promotes the necessary physical, chemical, and structural changes in the plasma membrane to facilitate release of acrosomal enzymes. (Because only sperm that have undergone capacitation are able to fertilize an egg, in IVF therapy the first stage of capacitation must be replicated in the laboratory prior to IVF if fertilization is to occur in the petri dish.)

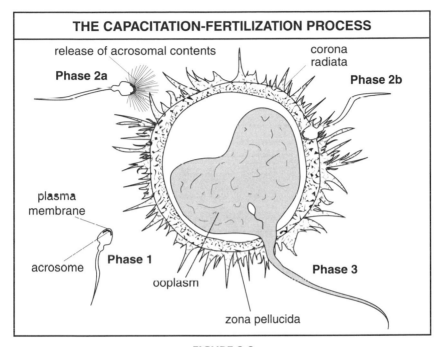

FIGURE 2-8

After the acrosome reaction has taken place, the successful sperm completes the fertilization process by burrowing through the zona pellucida and ooplasm to the nuclear material. The sperm sheds its body and tail upon penetration, and only the head (containing the genetic material) actually enters the egg. Figure 2-8 illustrates the following steps in the capacitation-fertilization process:

Phase 1: The plasma membrane fuses with the acrosome as the sperm pass into the reproductive tract to reach the egg, thus initiating capacitation.

Phase 2a: The acrosomal enzymes are released, and penetrate the cumulus mass cells of the egg.

Phase 2b: The acrosome fuses with the zona pellucida, thus completing capacitation.

Phase 3: The sperm burrows through the zona pellucida into the ooplasm of the egg.

The moment a sperm penetrates the egg's zona pellucida, a reaction in the egg fuses the zona and the perivitelline membrane into an impermeable shield that prevents other sperm from entering.

When fertilization occurs, the egg starts dividing within the zona covering, drawing its metabolic supplies from the ooplasm within the egg. Propelled by contractions of the fallopian tube, the dividing embryo begins its three- or four-day journey to the uterus and continues to divide after reaching it.

About two days after reaching the uterus, when the embryo has divided into more than 100 cells, it cracks open, and all the cells burst out through the fractured zona. This is known as *hatching.* These cells then try to burrow their way into the lining of the uterine wall. A portion of the growing embryo soon makes contact with the mother's circulatory system and becomes the earliest form of the *placenta,* from which the baby will receive its nourishment (see figure 2-9).

If an embryo implants anywhere but in the uterus, it is referred to as an *ectopic pregnancy.* In most cases, an ectopic pregnancy is due to embryonic implantation in the fallopian tube; this occurs about once in every 200 pregnancies. Isolated cases of implantation in the reproductive tract, such as on the ovary or elsewhere in the abdominal cavity, have been reported. In rare instances, such ectopic pregnancies have been known to develop to full term, but the baby invariably will not survive. (See chapter 9 for more information on ectopic pregnancies.)

Figure 2-9 follows the progress of an egg as it is ovulated from the follicle, becomes fertilized in the fallopian tube, and implants into the endometrium of the uterus. The dotted line plots the days that normally elapse as:

1. Ovulation occurs (and meiosis takes place prior to and during fertilization)
2. The fertilized egg, which has not yet divided, is now called a zygote

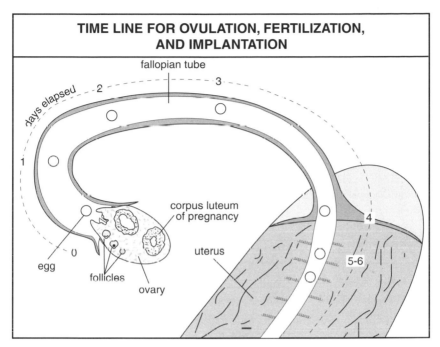

TIME LINE FOR OVULATION, FERTILIZATION, AND IMPLANTATION

FIGURE 2-9

3. The egg begins to divide and is now known as an embryo; at this point each *blastomere,* or cell, within the embryo is capable of developing into an identical embryo

4. The embryo develops into a mulberry-like structure known as a *morula*

5. A cavity develops within the embryo, which indicates the *blastocyst* stage

6. The process of *gastrulation* begins (cells are now dedicated to the development of specific embryonic layers that subsequently will form specific organs and structures; individual cells are no longer capable of developing into embryos)

At ovulation, the physical-chemical properties of the cervical mucus nurture the sperm as they pass through it, enhancing their quick passage and therefore capacitation as well. This is because hormonal changes around the time of ovulation ensure that the *microfibrilles,* or *myceles,* of the cervical mucus are arranged in a parallel manner. The sperm must then swim between the myceles in order to reach the uterus and, finally, the fallopian tubes. In addition, the cervical mucus becomes watery, and the amount produced (some of which may be discharged) increases significantly.

At another time during the menstrual cycle, the hormonal environment alters the arrangement of the myceles in the cervical mucus to form a barrier to the passage of sperm. During this time the mucus is thick, thus preventing the sperm from passing through the cervix.

The *Billings Method* of contraception is based on this phenomenon. A woman using the Billings Method predicts when she is likely to be ovulating by evaluating whether her cervical mucus is thick or watery. Because pregnancy can occur only around the time of ovulation, it is accordingly possible for her to identify the "safe period" when she is unlikely to conceive following unprotected intercourse.

HORMONES PREPARE THE BODY FOR CONCEPTION

Pregnancy, of course, begins with the fusion of the two gametes, but the preparations for conception begin long before fertilization occurs. The onset of puberty in both the man and the woman sets the stage for a biorhythmical hormonal orchestration that becomes more and more fine-tuned over the ensuing decade. It begins with the formation and release of hormones into the bloodstream, and the bodies of both sexes rely on a complex feedback mechanism to measure existing hormonal levels and determine when additional hormones should be released.

The *hypothalamus* (a small area in the midportion of the brain) and the *pituitary gland* (a small, grape-like structure that hangs from the base of the brain by a thin stalk) together regulate the formation and release of hormones. The hypothalamus, through its sensors, or *receptors,* constantly monitors female and male hormonal concentrations in the bloodstream and responds by regulating the release of small, proteinlike "messenger hormones" to the pituitary gland. These

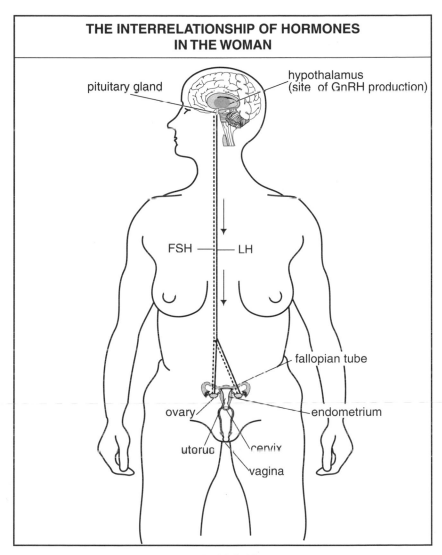

THE INTERRELATIONSHIP OF HORMONES
IN THE WOMAN

pituitary gland

hypothalamus
(site of GnRH production)

FSH ——|—— LH

fallopian tube

ovary

endometrium

uterus

cervix

vagina

FIGURE 2-10

messenger hormones are known as *gonadotropin-releasing hormones,*
or GnRH (see figure 2-10).

In response to the messenger hormones from the hypothalamus,
the pituitary gland determines the exact amount of hormones that it

in turn will release to stimulate the *gonads* (ovaries in the woman and testicles in the man). These hormones, or *gonadotropins,* are called *follicle-stimulating hormones* (FSH) and *luteinizing hormones* (LH). The hypothalamus closes the feedback circle by measuring the level of hormones produced by the gonads while at the same time monitoring the release of LH and FSH by the pituitary gland.

This "push-pull" interplay of messages and responses produces the cyclical hormonal environment in the woman that is designed solely to promote pregnancy. A "push-pull" mechanism also occurs in the man with regard to the release of *testosterone,* the male sex hormone. Similar feedback mechanisms regulate other hormonal responses in mammals, such as the functioning of the thyroid and adrenal glands.

There are two primary sex hormones in the female, *estrogen* and *progesterone;* in the male there is only one, testosterone. The pituitary gland releases identical hormones—FSH and LH—to the gonads of both the woman and the man, but the female and male gonads respond differently to these hormones. The level of female hormones fluctuates approximately monthly throughout the menstrual cycle, while male hormone production remains relatively constant.

In men, FSH and LH trigger the production of testosterone and influence the production and maturation of sperm. (The mechanism of male hormone production is not relevant to a proper understanding of IVF and will not be discussed in detail here.)

In women, extraneous factors as well as the level of circulating hormones and gonadotropins may influence the body's feedback mechanism. For example, the hypothalamus may be influenced by stress, pain, environmental changes, diseases in the woman's body, birth-control pills, and many forms of medication, including tranquilizers and blood-pressure medication.

The best way to understand this cyclical hormonal process is to trace the woman's hormonal pattern throughout a menstrual cycle. For practical purposes, the menstrual cycle will be considered to begin on the first day of menstruation. The following illustration is based on a 28-day menstrual cycle. However, it is important to remember that many women have somewhat shorter or longer menstrual cycles. In such cases, although the cyclic phases and ovulation occur in the manner described below, their length and timing vary according to the number of days in that particular cycle. For example, a woman with a cycle of 35 days is not likely to ovulate on day 14.

The First Half of the Cycle (the Follicular/ Proliferative Phase)

The body prepares for ovulation during the first two weeks of the menstrual cycle. During this two-week period, the lining of the uterus (endometrium) thickens or proliferates significantly and becomes very glandular under the influence of rising blood estrogen levels. This phase is accordingly often referred to as the *proliferative phase* of the cycle. Because this proliferation of the endometrium occurs at the same time as the development of the ovarian follicle(s), it is often also known as the *follicular phase*. From just prior to the beginning of the menstrual period until the middle of that cycle, the pituitary gland releases the gonadotropin FSH in ever-increasing amounts.

The release of FSH causes the formation of follicles in the ovaries as well as both the production of estrogen and the selection of eggs (usually one per follicle) that are to mature during that cycle. Often as many as 30 or even more follicles begin to develop under the stimulation of FSH, but in the natural cycle only one and sometimes two follicles progress to ovulation (see figure 2-11). The eggs that do not mature ultimately disintegrate and are absorbed into the ovary. This explains why so many eggs are lost during the reproductive life span, although a woman usually ovulates only one, sometimes two, and, very rarely, three eggs in any particular menstrual cycle.

Responding (usually at the middle of the menstrual cycle) to the rising estrogen levels in the bloodstream, the hypothalamus releases a surge of gonadotropin-releasing hormone (GnRH) when the estrogen reaches a critical level. This rush in GnRH production prompts the pituitary gland to produce a surge of LH, which had been released only in very low, erratic concentrations until this point. It is the sudden surge in LH that actually triggers ovulation.

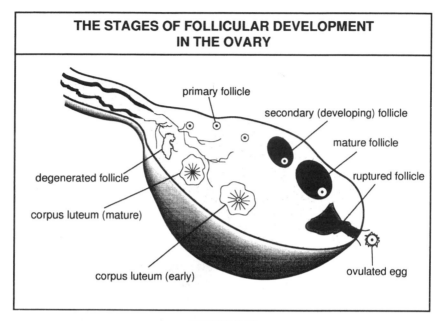

THE STAGES OF FOLLICULAR DEVELOPMENT IN THE OVARY

primary follicle

secondary (developing) follicle

mature follicle

ruptured follicle

degenerated follicle

corpus luteum (mature)

corpus luteum (early)

ovulated egg

FIGURE 2-11

Ovulation

At ovulation, a muscle connecting the ovary with the end of the fallopian tubes contracts, bringing the fimbriae closer to the follicle containing the egg. The fimbriae then gently massage and vacuum the follicle until the egg, which by this time is protruding from the follicle, is extruded. The fimbriae receive the egg and direct it into the fallopian tube, where contractions transport it toward the uterus.

The follicle collapses once the egg has been extruded and is transformed biochemically and hormonally. It takes on a yellowish color and is then referred to as the *corpus luteum* ("yellow body" in Latin).

All the while that the ovaries are nurturing eggs and producing hormones, the endometrium is developing in preparation for receiving an embryo. By the time ovulation occurs, it is about three times as thick as it was immediately after menstruation. (In chapter 8 we will discuss in detail the critical role the endometrium plays in successful implantation of the embryo.)

The Second Half of the Cycle (the Secretory/ Luteal Phase)

Once the corpus luteum forms, the ovary begins to secrete the hormone progesterone as well as estrogen, and the levels of progesterone begin to rise very rapidly. The progesterone converts the proliferated, glandular endometrium to a juicy structure capable of secreting nutrients that will sustain an embryo, hence the term *secretory phase.* The term *luteal phase* describes the stage of the menstrual cycle during which the corpus luteum produces the progesterone that enhances the secretory environment in the uterus.

The corpus luteum, through the production of both estrogen and progesterone, supports the survival of the secretory endometrium through the second half of the menstrual cycle. The life span of the corpus luteum is about 12 to 14 days if fertilization and implantation of the embryo into the endometrium do not occur. During that period the endometrium is sustained by the estrogen and progesterone produced by the corpus luteum. Once the corpus luteum begins to die, the hormonal support for the endometrium is lost, and two-thirds of it comes away (often with the unfertilized egg or unimplanted embryo) in the form of *menstruation.* (Figure 2-12 illustrates the relationship of hormone production to follicular and endometrial development throughout the menstrual cycle.)

Should the woman become pregnant, the hormone produced by the implanting embryo and the developing placenta, which is called *human chorionic gonadotropin,* or *hCG,* and has an effect similar to LH on the corpus luteum, prolongs the survival of the corpus luteum beyond its normal 12- to 14-day life span. The corpus luteum, in turn, continues to produce estrogen and progesterone to maintain the secretory environment of the endometrium, which nurtures the growth of the embryo before it makes contact with the blood system of the mother. Because the corpus luteum continues to exist and produces hormones that nurture the endometrium, the woman will miss her next menstrual period and should then suspect that she is pregnant.

The placenta begins to form as the developing embryo establishes a connection with the mother's system. The placenta is both the lifeline

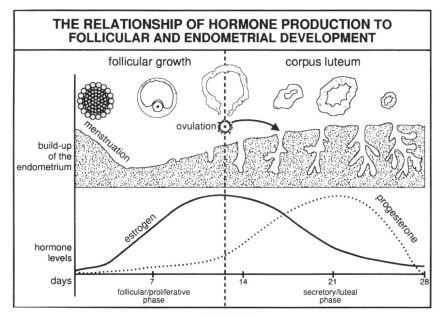

FIGURE 2-12

between the mother and baby's blood systems and the factory that nourishes the baby as pregnancy advances. Because the placenta is capable of producing estrogen and progesterone, it soon supplants the need for hormone production by the corpus luteum. The placenta itself supports the endometrium's survival after the 60th or 70th day following the last menstrual period. It has been proved that a pregnancy would continue after the 70th or 80th day even if both ovaries were removed because the placental hormones themselves are by then fully capable of sustaining the pregnancy.

After ovulation, the production of both LH and FSH declines significantly. If pregnancy does not occur, the hypothalamus begins to secrete more GnRH when the corpus luteum begins to die, thus initiating the next menstrual cycle. The same procedure is repeated over and over, with each hormonal cycle setting up the following one, much as each wave in the ocean sets up and determines the character and magnitude of the following wave. It is an indication of nature's ability to maintain biorhythms in a bewildering but organized fashion.

MISCARRIAGE IN EARLY PREGNANCY

Only about one out of every three embryos implants in the uterus long enough to delay the menstrual period. In other words, in two out of every three pregnancies the woman is not even aware that she has conceived.

Even when a pregnancy has been confirmed by a doctor, there is still a 16 to 20 percent chance of *miscarriage* (expelling of the products of conception after the death of the embryo/fetus) during the first three months of pregnancy. In most cases, the reason for this is not apparent; but in those situations where a reason is known, the vast majority of miscarriages are attributed to either a chromosomal abnormality in the developing offspring, immunologic factors affecting proper implantation, or hormonal insufficiency.

The use of sophisticated ultrasound techniques to confirm and monitor pregnancies has led to awareness of the phenomenon that not all embryos that implant in the uterus necessarily develop further. (*Ultrasound* is a painless diagnostic procedure that transforms high-frequency sound waves as they travel through body tissue and fluid into images on a TV-like screen. It enables the physician to clearly identify structures within the body and to guide instruments during certain procedures. There is no evidence that the ultrasound waves cause any damage.)

In some cases of confirmed multiple pregnancies, one (or more) of the implanted embryos are absorbed by the body or miscarried and passed through the vagina, thus reducing the number of surviving embryos. This spontaneous reduction in the number of pregnancies appears to be far more common than previously believed, even in those multiple pregnancies occurring without the use of fertility drugs.

An Abnormal Embryo

Early miscarriages usually occur because the embryo is abnormal. Miscarriage is nature's way of protecting the species from an inordinate number of abnormal offspring. These early miscarriages, which mostly occur even before the woman misses her period, are often referred to as *biochemical pregnancies* or *spontaneous menstrual abortions*.

The vast majority of such cases are the consequence of abnormal development in the mixing and replicating of the genetic blueprint. It has been shown that more than 70 percent of early pregnancy losses are attributable to a breakdown in the process of early mitosis and meiosis.

As a woman ages, meiosis and mitosis are far less likely to occur without problems, because an older woman's eggs are not able to divide or be fertilized as perfectly as those of a younger woman. This is why the babies of older women are more prone to Down syndrome and other chromosome abnormalities. (See chapter 8 for an explanation of how age impacts a woman's ability to have a healthy baby.)

Immunologic Factors

In some cases, the woman develops antibodies against the "root system" (trophoblast) of the implanting embryo (autoimmunity). In other cases, there is a rejection of the conceptus due to the sperm provider's immunologic makeup being too similar to that of the recipient (alloimmunity). (See chapter 8.)

Hormonal Insufficiency

In about 10 to 15 percent of all pregnancies, the embryo fails to implant because the amounts of hormones produced and the timing of their release were not perfectly synchronized. Such miscarriages, which may occur even if the embryo is perfect in every way, are attributed to *hormonal insufficiency.* This condition is caused by inadequate production of estrogen and/or progesterone during the menstrual cycle.

If hormonal insufficiency occurs because of abnormal hormonal production of estrogen during the follicular phase of the menstrual cycle, it is known as a *follicular phase insufficiency.* If attributable to inadequate production of hormones by the corpus luteum during the second phase of the cycle, it is referred to as a *luteal phase insufficiency.* Miscarriages due to follicular or luteal phase insufficiency may be associated with ovulation that occurs at the wrong time (either too late or too early), the production of inadequate amounts of hormones, an endometrium that responds inappropriately, or a combination of these factors.

Hormonal insufficiency may be perpetuated into early pregnancy, when the embryo is dependent on the survival of the corpus luteum before the placenta develops. Obviously, if implantation is imperfect because of improper hormonal stimulation, then *placentation* (the attachment of the placenta to the uterine wall) might also be defective. Poor placentation might prevent the baby from getting the proper nutrition. As a result, it might grow improperly and could be born too small or too early.

A pregnancy compromised by hormonal insufficiency may delay the onset of the anticipated menstrual period but then result in early miscarriage because of the inadequate hormonal environment. It is sometimes possible, however, to administer certain hormones in early pregnancy to sustain an embryo that otherwise would be lost.

Additional causes of miscarriage include thyroid and other hormonal irregularities, and kidney problems. It is believed that in addition to causing miscarriage, the misuse and abuse of narcotics, psychotropic drugs, alcohol, and nicotine during the first three months of pregnancy, when cell and organ differentiation are taking place, might significantly increase the incidence of birth defects as well as inhibit fetal growth and development.

It is likely that the thickness and quality of the endometrial lining as judged by ultrasound may also be an independent factor that affects the risk of miscarriage. We have come across a number of cases in which there was no apparent cause for recurrent spontaneous abortions (more than three), and the only determinant was that the endometrial lining appeared to be thinner than 9 mm.

It is the start in life that counts, and in most cases nature catches its mistakes. The high rate of embryo wastage and early miscarriage when conception occurs naturally may come as a surprise to many couples. However, it should provide a helpful perspective for couples who are considering comparable pregnancy rates offered by IVF and other options.

3

NATURAL CONCEPTION AND IVF:

TWO PATHWAYS TO PREGNANCY

Until relatively recently, pregnancy was not possible for couples who could not fulfill both requirements of conception: safe transport of the egg and sperm through the reproductive tract and fertilization within a supportive hormonal environment. IVF often solves this problem by bridging anatomical or physiologic disorders that until now have made pregnancy only an elusive dream for many couples.

CRITERIA FOR NATURAL CONCEPTION

There are five criteria a couple must meet in order for pregnancy to occur naturally:

1. Ovulation of a mature, healthy egg or eggs at the appropriate time, in association with the proper hormonal environment

2. Production of strong, healthy, mature sperm that are deposited in or adjacent to the woman's cervical canal around the time of ovulation

3. A physical-chemical environment that facilitates capacitation (activation) of the sperm as they pass through the woman's reproductive tract

4. A healthy fallopian tube that will promote the passage of sperm and eggs

5. A healthy uterine cavity with no abnormalities that might hinder implantation of the embryo, such as fibroid tumors (polyps that protrude into the cavity of the uterus) or scarring, and an endometrium that is thick enough and healthy enough to sustain an appropriate implantation in the uterus. This can be assessed by ultrasound evaluation of the endometrium prior to normal ovulation, by hormonal blood testing, and by a biopsy of the endometrium just prior to the menstrual period.

Couples who cannot fulfill all five criteria are unlikely to conceive or produce a healthy baby. The following section examines some of the ways in which common disease processes may prevent a couple from becoming pregnant. The remainder of this chapter explains how IVF can compensate for many of these deficiencies and thus enable a heretofore infertile couple to have a child.

ORGANIC AND PHYSIOLOGIC PROBLEMS THAT MAY PREVENT COUPLES FROM CONCEIVING NATURALLY

Neither sex contributes more heavily than the other to infertility problems. Roughly one-third of all infertile couples can trace their infertility to the woman, one-third to the man, and one-third to both partners.

Some Causes of Female Infertility

Organic *pelvic inflammatory disease* (PID) refers to the presence of structural damage in the woman's pelvis due to trauma, inflammation, tumors, congenital defects, or degenerative disease. The most common cause of infertility in a woman is damaged or blocked fallopian tubes that prevent the egg and sperm from uniting. Sexually transmitted diseases are a major cause of tubal scarring and blockage. In addition, scar tissue that forms after pelvic surgery may also lead to fertility problems.

Conditions such as *endometriosis,* in which the endometrium grows outside the uterus (causing scarring, pain, and heavy bleeding), can also damage the fallopian tubes and ovaries. The presence of even a minimal amount of endometriosis in the pelvis is believed to adversely affect fertility by releasing toxic substances that might reduce the potential of the egg to be fertilized. While the presence of minimal endometriosis might not necessarily adversely affect the passage of the egg from the ovary through the toxic environment to the fallopian tube, the toxins might diminish its ability to become fertilized. It has been shown that even the mildest form of endometriosis elicits a local immune response by releasing cells called *macrophages,* which wander through the pelvis and even into the fallopian tubes, destroying the eggs, sperm, and even the embryo. Accordingly, even the most minimal form of endometriosis may reduce fertility by as much as 70 percent through these mechanisms.

Damaged ovaries might also contribute to infertility. Sometimes an ovary cannot release an egg even though hormonal production is normal and the egg is adequately developed. It is also possible for an egg to be trapped within the follicle by scarring or thickening of the ovary's surface; this relatively rare condition may either be hereditary or induced by the malfunctioning of structures such as the adrenal gland.

More commonly, diseases such as PID or endometriosis, as well as surgically induced scarring, may anchor the ovaries in an awkward position or form a barrier that prevents the fimbriae from applying themselves properly to the ovaries' surface. Although one or both fallopian tubes may be perfectly free and mobile, the corresponding ovary could be inaccessible and unmovable. In such cases, the egg or eggs would be ovulated into the abdominal cavity instead of being retrieved by the fimbrae.

Abnormal ovulation is another cause for female infertility. Some women do not ovulate at all, while others ovulate too early or too late in their cycle for a pregnancy to occur. One of the reasons why normal fertility usually wanes after 35 is because ovulation is more likely to become abnormal later in the childbearing years.

In addition, it is believed that the quality of eggs decreases as women get older because the eggs' meiotic capacities are diminished by the aging process. The quality of the woman's eggs is one of the major determinants of whether a couple can get pregnant. (See chapter 8 for a detailed discussion of the effect of age on a woman's eggs.)

A woman may also be infertile because disease, surgery, or infection have damaged the lining of her uterus. Damage caused by scarring or the presence of tumors, such as fibroids, may prevent the embryo from attaching to the endometrium and developing properly.

Abnormalities in the size and shape of the uterus can also cause infertility problems. Sometimes women develop an abnormally shaped uterus as a result of exposure to certain drugs their mothers took during pregnancy. A classic example of this disorder is the "T-shaped" uterus and significantly smaller uterine cavity often found in women whose mothers took diethylstilbestrol (DES) during pregnancy.

Some women are unable to produce the cervical mucus that ensures the passage and vitality of the sperm. The production of hostile cervical mucus might be due to infection or abnormal physical and chemical properties in the secretions. Occasionally, surgery or injury to the cervix may have destroyed the glands that produce cervical secretions.

In some cases, women develop antibodies or an allergic response to their partner's sperm. These antibodies may be passed into the cervical secretions and thereby prevent fertilization by destroying or immobilizing the sperm.

(See chapter 9 for a more detailed discussion of the negative impacts of PID, endometriosis, DES exposure, and other conditions on a woman's fertility.)

Some Causes of Male Infertility

The causes of male infertility are often more difficult to define. Blockage of the sperm ducts is one obvious cause. Generalized blockage may be caused by sexually transmitted diseases. More easily identifiable blockage is caused by a *vasectomy* (voluntary surgery to occlude the sperm ducts for birth-control purposes). While it is usually possible to surgically reconnect the tubes after vasectomy, some men, especially those who underwent the procedure more than 10 years earlier, remain infertile because in the interim their systems have developed an immune reaction that results in the production of antibodies that destroy or immobilize their own sperm.

Another common cause of male infertility is a *varicocele,* a collection of dilated veins around the testicles that hinders sperm function by increasing body temperature in the scrotum. In order for the testicles to produce healthy sperm, the temperature in the scrotum must be lower than it is in the rest of the body.

Ideally, the testicles should have descended into the scrotum shortly after birth, but in some cases they do not reach the scrotum for years. In such circumstances it may be necessary to accomplish this surgically when the boy is very young to prevent the testicles from becoming severely damaged, thereby resulting in infertility. In rare cases, abnormal development of the testicles and/or sperm ducts may result from injury, disease, or hereditary abnormalities.

Certain drugs or chemicals in the environment may also inhibit sperm production and function. And as in women, drugs such as DES can produce abnormalities in the male offspring's reproductive system.

Finally, for reasons that are often not readily apparent, some men lack the adequate hormonal stimulation that is required for proper sperm production, or there is an abnormality in sperm parameters.

Unexplained Infertility

For about 10 percent of all infertile couples, the cause of the infertility cannot be readily determined by conventional diagnostic procedures. Such cases are referred to as "unexplained infertility." Modern IVF technology is making great strides in helping to identify some of the causes of so-called unexplained infertility. Improved testing techniques have made the causes of infertility easier to diagnose, and the majority of cases can now be diagnosed and generally are treatable. For example, many women initially diagnosed with "unexplained infertility" are ultimately found to have pelvic endometriosis that was not detected during laparoscopy (insertion through the abdomen of a lighted, telescope-like instrument that enables the physician to actually look inside the abdominal cavity) or laparotomy (see chapter 10 for a description of these procedures). For example, a condition called *nonpigmented endometriosis,* in which the endometrium may be growing inside the pelvic cavity with many of the same deleterious effects as overt endometriosis, cannot be detected by direct vision because no visible bleeding has occurred in these lesions. The fertility of these patients may be every bit as much compromised by these conditions as if they had detectable endometriosis. Simply stated, they turned out to have "undiagnosed" rather than "unexplained" infertility.

HOW IVF DIFFERS FROM NATURAL CONCEPTION

This section provides an overview of how IVF adapts the principles of human reproduction to achieve pregnancy. The procedures are described here in general terms and will be discussed in detail in subsequent chapters.

Fertility Drugs Are Used to Produce More Eggs

The administration of fertility drugs promotes the growth of more ovarian follicles than would develop naturally. These drugs also enable more follicles and eggs to mature instead of regressing prior to ovulation. Increasing the number of mature follicles facilitates the retrieval of more eggs and enhances the chance of creating more healthy embryos.

After reaching the uterus naturally, an embryo has approximately a 15 percent chance of surviving. With IVF, the implantation rate of a "good-quality" embryo or blastocyst, as determined microscopically and more recently through genetic expression of "competency" (see chapter 8, "Embryo Marker Expression Test [EMET]"), is about 20 and 40 percent respectively. To improve the chances of a successful IVF treatment, most programs transfer several embryos at one time into the uterus.

It may well be that when some women, especially those approaching menopause, are stimulated with fertility drugs, their ovaries, besides producing the eggs and the estrogen hormone that builds the endometrial lining, also might be producing disadvantageous chemicals and hormones that have an adverse effect on the lining. The problem is sidestepped in third-party parenting (ovum donation and gestational surrogacy) when the egg provider and the embryo recipient are not the same person.

The Chance of a Multiple Pregnancy Is Greater with IVF

While the success rate of an IVF procedure is directly related to the quality and number of embryos transferred to the woman's uterus, the more embryos transferred, the greater the risk of twins and high-order multiple pregnancies (triplets or greater). (See chapter 4 for a discussion of the risks of multiple pregnancies and the options available to couples.)

The risks of multiple babies is not simply a function of the number of embryos transferred but also embryo quality, which in turn is affected by egg quality. Older women who receive several embryos are far less likely to have multiple pregnancies than younger women receiving the same number of embryos. It is simply a question of embryo viability, which may not be detectable microscopically but might be an issue from a chromosomal point of view.

The impact of age on egg and embryo quality is an unalterable parameter that must be figured into the multiple-pregnancy equation. We have seen very few triplet pregnancies in women undergoing IVF over the age of 40, while the multiple pregnancy rate is at least twice as high in women under 35.

Eggs Are Retrieved from the Ovaries by Suction

Instead of waiting for the eggs to be ovulated naturally from the follicles, the IVF surgeon sucks them out of the ovaries through a long needle in a process known as *egg retrieval.* The needle can be inserted into the follicles through the vagina while the physician monitors its progress on an ultrasound screen (see chapter 6).

Prior to the advent of vaginal ultrasound egg retrievals, it was necessary to remove the eggs using a laparoscope inserted through an incision in the navel into the pelvic cavity, enabling the surgeon to see the pelvic organs and also to aspirate the eggs via a needle inserted through separate puncture sites in the lower abdomen. Laparoscopy is rarely performed for egg retrieval today.

Following retrieval, eggs are sent to the laboratory for fertilization. Egg retrieval is particularly appropriate when the fallopian tubes cannot retrieve or transport the eggs, when the woman is not able to ovulate properly, or in cases of unexplained infertility.

IVF Bypasses the Fallopian Tubes

The fallopian tubes are entirely bypassed in IVF because the eggs are retrieved directly from the ovaries and the fertilized embryos are transferred directly into the uterus via the vagina.

Sperm Are Partially Capacitated in the Laboratory Instead of in the Woman's Reproductive Tract

IVF eliminates many of the hurdles that sperm have to overcome, including escaping from the man's semen and passing through the cervical mucus. This is particularly important in cases where the man has an inadequate sperm count or poor sperm function. IVF is also helpful in situations when the woman forms cervical mucus that inadequately promotes capacitation or is hostile to the sperm. During IVF, laboratory procedures are substituted for the role of cervical mucus in capacitation, and the embryos are transferred directly into the uterus through a catheter to avoid exposure to hostile cervical mucus.

An IVF Embryo Is Not Likely to React to Either Partner's Antibodies

The body sometimes develops antibodies to sperm after it has become familiar with the spermatic blueprint. Accordingly, as sperm come into contact with bodily immune systems over time, women may build up sperm antibodies, and men may even develop antibodies to their own sperm.

IVF often evades fertility problems caused by antibodies produced by the woman and/or the man by enabling sperm to safely fertilize the eggs in the laboratory without interference from antibodies that would be present in the woman's reproductive tract. The resulting embryos are not affected by those antibodies because mammalian embryos do not have an immunological blueprint. In other words, embryos and fetuses are immunologically inert prior to birth. Thus, the woman's body, which might produce antibodies against sperm, tolerates the embryo because it is an unfamiliar, immunologically inert structure against which her body has not yet developed antibodies.

IVF Is Both a Treatment and a Diagnostic Procedure

IVF has a built-in diagnostic capability unmatched in nature or by any other method of evaluating or treating infertility. In ideal circumstances there is a 70 percent or greater chance that any one egg will fertilize in the laboratory. This affords the couple a chance to see whether they are capable of achieving fertilization together. IVF technology has brought to light many instances in which a woman's egg cannot be fertilized by her partner's sperm and sometimes not by any sperm. The reason for this is not always readily identifiable; the problem could lie with the egg, the sperm, or both. If several mature eggs fail to fertilize, this information can help couples make important decisions regarding their future plans. Although the test is not 100 percent foolproof, failed fertilization should encourage couples to consider micromanipulation, the use of donor eggs, donor sperm, donor embryos, or adoption (see chapters 11 and 14). No other method of treating infertility enables a physician to reach this diagnostic conclusion. IVF might be called the ultimate fertility test.

Another diagnostic application of IVF would be when, for no readily apparent reason, the fallopian tubes might be unable to properly receive and/or transport the egg, sperm, and embryos. Because IVF by its very nature bypasses the fallopian tubes, it might, through a process of exclusion, offer an answer and/or a solution to this problem.

IVF Requires a Heavy Emotional, Physical, and Financial Investment

The most significant difference between IVF and natural pregnancy is that a couple must sacrifice a great deal of their personal privacy before and during the IVF procedure, whereas natural conception is a private matter. An IVF couple must bare some of their deepest secrets and fears to the clinic staff and allow themselves to be manipulated physically and emotionally as they progress through the procedure. In addition, IVF is inordinately expensive—and there is no second prize if a woman does not conceive following the procedure. The couple will not have another chance at IVF pregnancy without making the same emotional, physical, and financial commitment again. In natural conception there's always next month, and the following month, and hope for the future, without the major costs that IVF exacts.

DOES IVF INCREASE THE RISK OF BIRTH DEFECTS?

In spite of several reports suggesting that IVF babies are more likely to be born with birth defects, there is little evidence to support the implication that the technique of IVF itself increases this risk. Certainly, with more and more women postponing childbearing to a later age and more and more men with sperm dysfunction resorting to IVF, the effect of the woman's age and the increased incidence of sperm chromosomal abnormalities associated with male infertility could increase the risk of both miscarriages and birth defects. However, short of remaining childless, what other recourse would couples with such forms of infertility have other than to resort to IVF?

CHAPTER

4

IVF STEP 1:

PREPARATION FOR
TREATMENT

Most IVF procedures are based on some variation of the following steps: (1) preparation for treatment, (2) induction of ovulation, (3) egg retrieval, and (4) embryo transfer. All successful IVF programs must be highly organized and exquisitely timed, just as in nature the fertilization process is organized and timed.

Each of these four basic steps in an IVF treatment cycle should be regarded as a hurdle that a couple must overcome before proceeding further. (The term *treatment cycle* refers to the menstrual cycle during which a particular IVF procedure is performed.) Occasionally, a couple may successfully negotiate one hurdle but then be unable to surmount the next step, in which case they would usually begin the treatment cycle anew after allowing the woman's body to rest for a month or two. In general, a couple's chances for successful IVF increase as they put each hurdle behind them.

The descriptions of IVF procedures in chapters 4 through 7 have been designed to provide an overview of what an infertile couple might expect to experience physically and emotionally during the treatment cycle. Because a truly comprehensive IVF program responds to—and often anticipates—the couple's emotional needs throughout the treatment cycle, some of the techniques that an IVF program might use to address emotional needs are included in the description of clinical procedures. We do not mean to imply that any of these scenarios is the best or the only way that IVF should be performed.

ACCEPTANCE INTO AN IVF PROGRAM

Before being admitted into any IVF program, the couple would probably be required to have a complete medical evaluation. They would most likely undergo all the routine steps of an infertility assessment, usually performed by their own primary physician, in order to rule out the possibility that procedures other than IVF might better address their needs.

The couple would probably be required to forward their medical records to the IVF program and are likely to be asked to provide additional background. They should expect to be encouraged to speak frankly about themselves and their personal habits (including their sexual practices, use and abuse of recreational drugs, general lifestyle, and other parameters that are known to impact fertility). In many programs, the couple also would undergo psychological counseling. Following a thorough evaluation of the materials submitted by the couple and their primary physician, the medical staff would then decide whether the couple is eligible for IVF.

Once accepted into the program, the couple would probably undergo orientation, including an explanation of the emotional, physical, and financial commitments that IVF would require. The orientation process could take place through letters, other written material, e-mail, and/or by telephone. It may also take place on site if the couple are able to visit the clinic prior to commencement of the treatment cycle.

In some ART programs the couple have to be at the clinic during the entire process, including *induction of ovulation* (usually a series of daily injections of fertility drugs). In other programs, couples are encouraged to initiate the induction of ovulation with their own gynecologist and are required to be on site only for the last few days of the cycle prior to egg retrieval and embryo transfer.

ORGANIZATION OF A TYPICAL IVF PROGRAM

In many programs, one or more clinical coordinators play an important role in assisting the physician to ensure that the couple receive proper emotional preparation throughout the process. The clinical coordinator plays a central role and administers many treatment procedures that have previously been agreed upon by the entire medical staff.

In such a coordinator-oriented program, the couple could anticipate spending as much if not more time with a clinical coordinator as with the physician. This is because a clinical coordinator usually functions as the couple's advocate—the liaison between the couple and all the other members of the IVF team, including the physician. However, this is not meant to imply that both the clinical and administrative roles could not be fulfilled by a physician who has a personality and attitude that engenders a feeling of well-being, relaxation, and optimism. In general, though, clinical coordinators contribute significantly to the smooth operation of many IVF programs.

It is the responsibility of the person who guides the couple throughout the treatment cycle, whether that is physician or clinical coordinator, to explain every step along the way so the couple know exactly what to expect. In addition, the same staff member who is responsible for establishing the initial rapport with the couple should be their contact person throughout their tenure with the program.

In most programs the couple will be introduced to the staff, taken on a tour of the facility, and encouraged to ask a lot of questions. The staff in an IVF program, including the clerical personnel, should be upbeat and encouraging when they deal with infertile couples. The empathic IVF program will provide a relaxing, low-key environment that offers subtle support to both partners during their time of emotional need. Although the couple should be well aware that no program can guarantee a pregnancy, even after several attempts, a congenial atmosphere fostered by the staff should help both partners maintain a mood of guarded optimism.

Some IVF programs provide access to a nurse-counselor with special expertise in the psychological aspects of infertility. Although the participation of a nurse-counselor is not essential in order for a couple to conceive, an IVF team member who can predict the way a couple might react, and therefore help improve their tolerance to the emotional roller-coaster ride of IVF, adds another dimension of caring to the program.

TESTS THAT MAY BE CONDUCTED PRIOR TO IVF

Before the couple has a pretreatment consultation with the physician, it is likely that the partners will be asked to complete some or all of the following tests. (See chapter 10 for a detailed explanation of most of the tests listed in this chapter as well as others the couple might undergo prior to IVF.)

Tests for Certain Viral Infections

The HIV/AIDS test.   A couple should defer pregnancy until they are sure that neither partner carries a disease that can seriously prejudice the health, well-being, and even the survival of the offspring. Although this is a personal decision to be resolved between the man and the woman, the physician enters the picture when IVF is being considered. As the catalyst responsible for creating the circumstances under which a new life might be conceived, the physician has a medical, legal, and moral obligation to make every attempt to ensure that IVF does not lead to the birth of a child who suffers from a life-endangering disease such as *acquired immunodeficiency syndrome* (AIDS).

Accordingly, many programs require that an HIV (human immunodeficiency virus; the virus that causes AIDS) test be done on both partners prior to any IVF procedure. Unfortunately, this test still does not completely rule out the presence of HIV infection because a person may not register positive for up to six months after infection by HIV. However, the test does provide a good screen to help protect an IVF program from being instrumental in the birth of damaged offspring. (Another reason for administering the HIV test to all new patients is to protect medical and laboratory personnel who work with the couple.)

Some physicians also test both partners for HIV before the woman undergoes any treatment to enhance fertility, such as reconstructive tubal surgery. This is because if one of the partners is HIV-positive and a baby with HIV is born after successful tubal surgery, the couple might argue that they would not have consented to treatment had they known they could transmit HIV to a baby.

We recognize that the decision to undergo HIV testing is a very personal one and that a physician certainly cannot force anyone to have this test. Nevertheless, we strongly advise that the issue be discussed prior to initiating treatment for infertility.

Some IVF couples have expressed concern that HIV might be transmitted through fertility drugs because some of these drugs (e.g., those produced by Repronex, Bravelle-Ferring Pharmaceuticals, and Pergonal-Serono Laboratories) are derived from the urine of menopausal women. Most experts agree, however, that HIV does not survive the purification and extraction process to which these drugs are subjected. (See "Cryopreservation as an Option" in chapter 15 for further discussion about protection against HIV/AIDS.) Moreover, most of the gonadotropins administered today are genetically engineered products that are free of viral contamination.

Hepatitis B and C infection.   Hepatitis B and C, which may be transmitted sexually or through blood, may also be transmitted from an infected mother to her *conceptus* (the collective term for the embryo, as well as the developing fetus and its placenta). Women who test positive for either of these viruses should be counseled that the risk of transmission could be as high as 10 percent and that many fetuses so infected may succumb, be born with liver damage, or acquire serious congenital abnormalities. Additionally, there is a slight possibility that fertilization of eggs with sperm derived from a man who tests positive will infect the embryo and similarly place the fetus at risk. Since active infection with hepatitis B and C (or a carrier state) is difficult and often impossible to eradicate, couples/individuals so infected often choose to take a calculated risk and proceed with fertility treatment. However, it is incumbent upon the treating physician to relay all relevant information that spells out such risk, so that patients can make a well-informed decision before proceeding.

Syphilis. The incidence of venereal infection with syphilis is on the rise throughout the world. While active infection with this organism will usually not prevent fertilization, it can cause serious congenital abnormalities in the offspring. Thus all men and women undergoing IVF should have their blood tested for syphilis and, if detected, be treated before proceeding with IVF.

Chlamydia and gonorrhea. Infection of the male and/or female partner with chlamydia or gonorrhea is not transmitted to the offspring. However, since these diseases are sexually transmitted and result in major health problems, all parties undergoing fertility treatment should be tested. (See chapter 9 for a discussion of the impacts of chlamydia on infertility.)

Ureaplasma urealyticum. Ureaplasma is a microorganism that occurs in the reproductive tracts of both sexes and may interfere with sperm transport and/or embryo implantation. It commonly produces no symptoms in either partner. When present in the cervical secretions, it can be transmitted to the uterine cavity during embryo transfer, where it might interfere with implantation. Ideally, the male partner should also be cultured for ureaplasma. If the organism is found in either partner, both should be treated concurrently with the appropriate antibiotic.

Sperm Quality

In any IVF program the male partner will almost certainly be asked to submit to a basic semen analysis. The purpose is twofold: (1) to ensure that the sperm's viability and mobility are not abnormal and/or have not changed significantly since the last sperm assessment, which would dramatically affect the couple's rational expectations for successful IVF; and (2) to protect the program from medical-legal liability in case the man has developed an undetected fertility problem since his sperm were last evaluated. The quality of the sperm, along with the age of the woman undergoing egg retrieval, are the two most important factors that enable the physician to predict the likelihood of the couple getting pregnant through IVF.

Sperm DNA Integrity Assay (SDIA)

Over the last few years it has become known that certain abnormalities in sperm DNA can thwart attempts to achieve a viable pregnancy even in cases where the man has normal sperm parameters. The development of tests such as the *sperm DNA integrity assay* (SDIA) hold great promise for couples who otherwise might have unexplained infertility, IVF failure, or pregnancy loss. Many women do conceive in spite of their partners' abnormal SDIA and give birth to healthy babies. However, an abnormal SDIA markedly reduces the pregnancy rate, increases the risk of first-trimester miscarriages, and reduces the natural as well as the ART birthrate. It is important to point out that an abnormal SDIA neither results in structural or numerical chromosome abnormalities of the embryo nor impairs fertilization potential or appearance of the embryo.

Sperm Antibody Tests

More and more programs require that the male partner take a sperm test to determine whether he is harboring sperm antibodies, which could affect the ability of his sperm to fertilize an egg and thereby adversely affect the chances of a successful outcome with IVF. Moreover, the presence of sperm antibodies in the man will significantly influence the manner in which sperm is prepared for the IVF process. In some cases, the presence of high concentrations of sperm antibodies could mandate the performance of *intracytoplasmic sperm injection* (ICSI), where a single sperm is captured in a thin glass needle and injected directly into the egg to promote fertilization, thus avoiding the antibodies.

Pelvic Measurement

A careful pelvic examination is important in order to evaluate for the presence of irregularities in the contour of the uterus or the adjacent pelvic organs. Their presence might suggest the existence of fibroid tumors, ovarian cysts, swollen fallopian tubes, and other conditions that might affect treatment.

Uterine Measurement (Mock Embryo Transfer)

The introduction of ultrasound-guided embryo transfer has made it possible to place the embryos accurately about 1 cm below the roof of the uterine cavity. However, it is not always possible to accurately identify the location of the roof of the uterine cavity or the tip of the flexible embryo-transfer catheter as it is introduced into the uterine cavity. This is especially the case when the uterus is enlarged, has fibroid tumors or adenomyosis, and/or is tipped backwards (severely retroverted). Accordingly, it is very helpful to have premeasured the uterine depth before undertaking an embryo transfer. At the time of pelvic examination a probe or a embryo-transfer catheter may be introduced via the cervix into the uterine cavity to determine the exact depth of the uterus in order to ensure proper placement of the catheter at the time of embryo transfer. The relative ease or difficulty with which the embryo-transfer catheter is introduced will also assist in planning strategy for the embryo-transfer procedure.

Fluid Ultrasonography (FUS) or Hysteroscopy

We routinely perform *fluid ultrasonography* (FUS) or *hysteroscopy* on women scheduled for IVF if the woman has not undergone the examination for a year or two. FUS involves the injection of a liquid into the uterus via the cervix, allowing ultrasound examination of the uterus and fallopian tubes. Hysteroscopy is the examination of the cervix and inside of the uterus for defects by means of a lighted, telescope-like instrument that is passed through the cervix into the uterus.

FUS or hysteroscopy is not required in cases where the woman has had a hysteroscopy within 18 months in which the uterine cavity was shown to be normal. We would perform FUS or hysteroscopy in cases where a *hysterosalpingogram* or the advent of disease/symptoms suggest the presence of surface lesions in the uterine cavity might have occurred after a prior FUS or hysteroscopy was performed. In one out of eight cases, surface lesions that might interfere with implantation are detected by the routine performance of FUS or hysteroscopy; these should be treated before the woman undergoes IVF. This often occurs despite the fact that a recent hysterosalpingogram was reported as being normal and/or that the woman shows no evidence of disease.

FUS and hysteroscopy can easily be performed in the doctor's office and do not require any significant postoperative care. We have found this approach to be well received by our patients and are convinced that the routine implementation of FUS or hysteroscopy followed by appropriate treatment, when indicated, has prevented numerous women from undergoing otherwise futile attempts at IVF.

Measurement of FSH, Estradiol, and Inhibin B Blood Levels

The measurement of the hormones FSH, *blood estradiol* (the concentration of estrogen in the woman's blood, also known as E_2), and Inhibin B on the third day of a menstrual cycle preceding IVF helps evaluate the potential ability of the woman's ovaries to respond to fertility drugs. It also provides information that the physician can use to select the ideal dosage and regimen of fertility drugs to achieve an optimal response. For this reason, these hormones should be measured in all regularly menstruating women scheduled to undergo IVF. An FSH level of 9.0 miu/ml or greater in association with a blood estradiol level of less than 70 pg/ml, as well as an Inhibin B blood level of less than 45 ng/ml is predictive of incipient *ovarian failure* (resistance to stimulation with fertility drugs).

Immunologic Testing

In certain types of female infertility, the embryo fails to attach properly to the endometrial lining because of immunologic problems. In such cases the woman most often loses the pregnancy so early that she does not even know she was pregnant. In reality, this is better described as a "mini-miscarriage" rather than infertility. The performance of certain immunologic tests, including, but not limited to, an antiphospholipid antibody panel (APA), antithyroid antibody (ATA) panel, natural killer cell cytotoxicity/activity (NKa) test, and reproductive immunophenotype (RIP), will assist in diagnosing this relatively common cause of infertility, miscarriage, and IVF failure (see chapter 8).

Measurement of Prolactin

A markedly raised blood prolactin level might interfere with both endometrial proliferation and follicle growth and development, thereby reducing the likelihood of a successful pregnancy. Blood prolactin levels might be raised as a consequence of a prolactin-producing pituitary tumor or other intracranial lesions. In addition, the use of certain drugs, such as tranquilizers, ganglion blocker antihypertensives, antidepressants, thyiazides, and narcotics, can elevate the blood prolactin level. Another important consideration is that mild to moderately raised prolactin levels often present as one of the earliest signs of an impending or existing hypothyroid state, often with high-normal levels of blood *thyroid-stimulating hormone* (TSH) and usually associated with the presence of ATA detectible in the blood. The presence of ATA, in turn, will in 50 percent of cases point to an underlying failure of embryos to attach properly to the uterine wall, resulting in *immunologic implantation failure.*

Antral Follicle Count (AFC)

The performance of an *antral follicle count* (AFC), or ultrasound examination of the ovaries, during the first few days of the menstrual cycle will reveal the presence of small antral (fluid-filled) follicles. It is these follicles that can ultimately develop into large egg-bearing follicles with ovarian stimulation. The number of antral follicles suggests the potential number of eggs that could become available for egg retrieval under optimal circumstances.

THE PRETREATMENT CONSULTATION

Once the appropriate tests have been completed, the physician and per-haps the clinical coordinator will discuss with the couple what to expect throughout the treatment cycle. Although the couple may have a general idea, the physician will reinforce what they have already been told and will encourage them to ask questions.

The physician probably will also outline some of the decisions the couple will have to make in the next few days. These include (1) how many eggs they wish to have fertilized, (2) what they want to do with any excess eggs, (3) how many embryos they want to have transferred into the uterus, (4) how they wish to dispose of any excess embryos (i.e., through embryo cryopreservation, also known as freezing, or donation), and (5) how they would deal with a high-order multiple pregnancy. Although these questions do not all have to be answered at the same time, the physician will probably touch on all of the relevant issues during this consultation in order to give the couple ample time to make their decision.

Preparing for the Inevitable Trade-off: The Probability of Pregnancy vs. the Risk of High-Order Multiple Births

Because an embryo's average chance of implanting is about 20 percent with conventional IVF, enough embryos must be transferred into the uterus to ensure the highest probable birthrate. It has been our experi-ence at SIRM that in women under 40 with a well-prepared endometri-um and with good-quality embryos, placement of three embryos or two blastocysts (embryos that are two to three days older) into the uterus yields about a 40 percent chance of having a baby. (See chapter 8 for a discussion about the technique and advisability of transferring blastocysts into the woman's uterus).

However, the couple wishing to maximize their chances of pregnan-cy by increasing the number of embryos transferred must be prepared to confront the unavoidable tradeoff: The more embryos, the greater the risk of multiple births. The multiple-pregnancy rate from IVF in women under 40 is twins in about one out of every three and triplets or greater (high-order multiple pregnancy) in about one out of every 20 pregnancies.

The physician should explain that it is the number of *viable* embryos transferred to the uterus rather than the absolute number (whether or not they are known to be viable) that determines the risk of multiple gestation. Accordingly, the older patient undergoing IVF will likely be advised to have more embryos transferred than would be the case with her younger counterpart. This is because the risk of multiple pregnancies has more to do with the number of viable embryos than with the absolute number transferred. The number of embryos transferred, therefore, should be influenced by the woman's age.

The risks associated with a high-order multiple pregnancy. The couple must be thoroughly educated on the implications of a high-order multiple pregnancy (triplets or greater) before they decide how many embryos to have transferred. While most women can tolerate a twin pregnancy, a higher-order multiple pregnancy threatens the well-being of both mother and babies. Moreover, the risks become greater to both mother and babies as the number of fetuses increases.

Risks to the mother that are especially acute during a high-order multiple pregnancy include high blood pressure, uterine bleeding, and problems associated with a cesarean section. (The incidence of cesarean sections increases dramatically in multiple pregnancies.)

The primary threat to the physical and intellectual well-being of the babies stems from complications resulting from premature birth. Multiple births often occur prematurely, and the more babies, the more premature their birth. Prematurity can cause one or possibly all of the babies to be born brain-damaged and/or with a dangerously low birth weight that can endanger their survival.

Selective reduction of pregnancy. Because of the serious complications that so often occur in high-order multiple pregnancies, most IVF programs tend to transfer fewer embryos or blastocysts to the uterus than was the case a few years ago and counsel couples on the concept of selectively reducing the size of a multiple pregnancy as a possible lifesaving measure for the remaining fetuses.

Selective reduction of pregnancy, which is usually performed prior to completion of the third month of gestation, involves the injection of a chemical under guidance by ultrasound directly into one or more developing fetuses. This causes the involved fetus(es) to succumb almost immediately and be absorbed by the body. Selective reduction of pregnancy can cause a miscarriage in the remaining fetus(es), but this occurs infrequently when the procedure is done by an expert. Experience has demonstrated that the risk of complete miscarriage or damage to the remaining fetuses is very small in cases where the fetuses are not *identical* (from the same embryo), as is virtually always the case with a multiple pregnancy following IVF. This is because IVF multiple pregnancies are almost always *fraternal* (from different embryos), having separate placentas and hence separate blood supplies.

We at SIRM advocate against women carrying more than two babies and advise receptive patients to reduce triplets to twins. We would definitely not suggest selective reduction in cases where there are fewer than three babies in the uterus unless indicated by unusual medical circumstances, such as one of twins being affected by a serious genetic/chromosomal defect.

IVF might be considered a pro-life procedure because by its very nature it is the opposite of abortion. Yet many physicians who perform IVF strongly believe that selective termination of pregnancy in the interest of saving life is acceptable or at least presents a possible option. We believe that couples should always be made aware, in an unbiased manner, of the option of selective termination of pregnancy in a pro-choice environment.

Constructing a framework for decision making. Before the couple can decide how many eggs should be fertilized, they first have to decide whether they are willing to risk a high-order multiple pregnancy. At this point, the physician might say to them:

There is a difference of opinion as to how many embryos should be transferred into the uterus. What you need to remember is that there is a trade-off. If you put in more embryos you have a higher chance of pregnancy, but also a greater chance of a high-order multiple pregnancy (triplets or greater), and this can be dangerous for the mother and the babies. We have found that where the egg provider is 35 to 40 years old, two embryos is a safe number to transfer to the uterus. In women over 40, three embryos can reasonably be transferred to the uterus with a relatively low expectation of high-order multiple pregnancies.

At SIRM we tend to *cryopreserve* (freeze and store) all remaining (non-transferred) embryos/blastocysts deemed to be viable. In most cases, the embryos are first kept in culture for an additional two to three days, and only those that develop into good-quality blastocysts are frozen and stored. In this way, upon transferring thawed blastocysts in a subsequent cycle, we are able to achieve good pregnancy rates.

5

IVF STEP 2:

INDUCTION OF OVULATION

A woman undergoing IVF is given fertility drugs for two reasons: (1) to control the timing of ovulation so the eggs can be retrieved before they are ovulated and (2) to promote the growth and development of an optimal number of ovarian follicles in order to allow the woman to produce as many fully developed mature eggs as possible. IVF may also be performed in natural cycles (cycles in which no fertility drugs are administered); however, this can only be done in cases where the woman is ovulating normally. The success rate with natural-cycle IVF is much lower because in such cases it is unlikely that more than one or two eggs can be retrieved at a time.

The ovulation of more than one egg that has been induced through the administration of fertility drugs is known as *superovulation*. The term *controlled ovarian hyperstimulation* (COH) encompasses the concept of deliberate induction of superovulation but also refers to production of an exaggerated hormonal response that favors the growth, development, and maturation of multiple ovarian follicles and eggs. The terms *stimulation, superovulation,* and *controlled ovarian hyperstimulation* are often used interchangeably. *Folliculogenesis* is the process of follicle growth and development.

The development of the eggs in the woman's ovaries is measured by the concentration of the estradiol (the hormone estrogen secreted into the bloodstream by the growing ovarian follicles) in her blood and/or measurement of the developing follicles by ultrasound. It has been shown that the greater the degree of stimulation, the more eggs will be available for retrieval.

Ovulation can be expected to occur about 38 to 42 hours after a woman is optimally stimulated. Egg retrieval, therefore, has to be scheduled for a few hours prior to the anticipated time of ovulation so the eggs can be retrieved *before* being expelled into the abdominal cavity. As will be explained later, the methods of inducing ovulation, assessing the degree of stimulation, and predicting the time of ovulation vary according to the fertility drug used.

Induction of ovulation makes physical and emotional demands on the couple. The woman should expect to undergo daily administration of a fertility drug, usually by injection, as well as blood tests and/or ultrasound evaluations to monitor her progress. In addition, both partners should be prepared to cope with the strong emotions that some women experience because of the hormonal changes introduced by the fertility drugs. As one clinical coordinator explained:

It doesn't take anything to make women emotional at this point. I have at least one patient a week sobbing in my office just looking at the plants. Sometimes they will even cry over dog-food commercials. The couple has to be prepared for this, and the man should be especially supportive and tolerant.

FERTILITY DRUG THERAPIES

The following section outlines the most common fertility drugs used in the United States. In general, the woman's response to these drugs will depend on her pattern of ovulation and her age.

Clomiphene Citrate

Clomiphene citrate is the most popular method of inducing ovulation and in the 1980s was the most widely used method for COH in preparation for IVF. It is a synthetic hormone that deceives the hypothalamus into thinking that the body's estrogen level is too low. In response, the hypothalamus releases GnRH (gonadotropin-releasing hormone), which in turn prompts the pituitary gland to release an increased amount of FSH (follicle-stimulating hormone). As happens in nature, the increased secretion of FSH stimulates development of the follicles, ultimately resulting in ovulation. The growing follicles secrete estrogen into the bloodstream, thus closing the feedback circle that the hypothalamus initiated in response to the anti-estrogen properties of clomiphene citrate. (When marketed in the United States, clomiphene is also known as Clomid and Serophene.)

The administration of clomiphene citrate enhances the normal cyclical pattern of follicular development and ovulation. If initiated as early as day 2 or day 3 of the menstrual cycle, it usually induces ovulation on day 13 or 14 of a regular 28-day cycle. If administered later, such as on day 5, ovulation could occur as late as day 16 or 17, and the length of the cycle may be extended. If the woman does not stimulate appropriately on the original dosage of clomiphene, the dosage may be increased to achieve optimal stimulation.

We sometimes administer hCG (human chorionic gonadotropin) to the woman once ultrasound examinations and hormonal evaluations confirm optimal follicular development. In such cases, ovulation will usually occur about 38 hours later.

The prolonged usage of clomiphene for more than three consecutive cycles may lead to the accumulation of one of its components (*zuclomiphene*), which will reduce the amount and alter the quality of the cervical mucus, with negative implications for the passage and capacitation of the sperm. It is also likely to thin the uterine lining and thereby reduce the chances of a healthy implantation. This is the reason why the prolonged usage of clomiphene without at least one month's break every three months is associated with reduced pregnancy rates and a much higher rate of spontaneous abortion, should pregnancy occur. It also explains why 80 percent of births that occur following the use of clomiphene are conceived during the first three months of stimulation and why hardly any pregnancies occur at all in women who have taken clomiphene more than five or six months without a break. One month's hiatus is sufficient to allow for the elimination of zuclomiphene from the body and will restore the potential to respond optimally to clomiphene.

It has been observed that few women as they get older show a declining response to clomiphene. However, in spite of the fact that they appear to ovulate on chlomiphene treatment, they frequently develop poor mucus and a poor endometrial lining from the inception of clomiphene administration. We accordingly believe that clomiphene should rarely be prescribed to women over the age of 35 and is relatively contraindicated for women over 40.

Two major advantages of clomiphene are its relatively low cost and the fact that it can be taken orally instead of by injection. A distinct disadvantage is that when administered alone it does not stimulate the growth and maturation of as many follicles as do alternative therapies such as gonadotropins (Follistim, Gonal F, Repronex, Bravelle) or clomiphene plus gonadotropins; accordingly, fewer eggs can be retrieved.

Side effects of clomiphene citrate.   The side effects associated with clomiphene citrate are related to the follicular development this drug stimulates. When administered alone, a *luteal-phase defect* (inadequate production of progesterone by the corpus luteum to sustain the endometrium) may result if the follicles do not develop properly. This would hinder implantation by preventing the endometrium from responding optimally to the progesterone produced by the corpus luteum. In about 15 percent of clomiphene-treated cycles the hormonal changes associated with ovulation take place along with the commensurate rise in blood progesterone level, but the egg is *not* released. This form of "trapped ovulation" is referred to as *luteinized unruptured follicle syndrome* (LUFS). Clomiphene may also interfere with the nurturing effect estrogen must have on the developing endometrium. In addition, traces of clomiphene that might linger in the woman's circulatory system for many weeks may inhibit the normal function of enzymes produced by the developing follicular cells.

Too high a dose of clomiphene may cause follicles to grow too rapidly, producing large fluid-filled collections known as *cysts*. This may lead to tenderness and swelling of the ovaries, visual disturbances, and hot flashes similar to those at menopause.

Finally, too high a dose of clomiphene may decrease the amount of cervical mucus produced and may also reduce its quality, with negative implications for the passage and capacitation of the sperm. Too high a dosage may also decrease the thickness of the uterine lining.

Safety of clomiphene citrate.   Some studies have suggested that clomiphene citrate has caused birth defects or a higher miscarriage rate in laboratory animals and could, therefore, potentially threaten human offspring. Other studies have suggested that clomiphene administered for more than 12 sequential months increases the subsequent risk of ovarian cancer. However, if clomiphene is administered appropriately and is taken under proper supervision, it is a safe and effective method for induction of ovulation.

The fear that clomiphene might cause birth defects arises from the fact that its inner structure, or nucleus, is very similar to that of the hormone DES (diethylstilbestrol), which is known to have caused so many birth defects when administered to pregnant women. Although it is theoretically possible that clomiphene might cause such defects, birth statistics do not indicate an increased birth-defect rate after stimulation with the drug. The laboratory studies mentioned above should not be ignored, however, but should be heeded as a guide to safe, prudent administration of fertility drugs.

Since it is not known with certainty whether clomiphene citrate might adversely affect the developing fetus, we caution that this agent should be taken only when it is absolutely certain that the woman is not pregnant. The appearance of a menstrual period does not provide adequate certainty, because more than 10 percent of women might bleed during early pregnancy. Assessment by a physician, or even a home pregnancy test, provides greater assurance that a pregnancy does not exist.

The administration of clomiphene as a fertility agent over a series of months might promote ovulatory problems. It has been observed that in one out of five cases where clomiphene is administered, the egg remains trapped in the follicle after ovulation. Therefore, the practice of physicians saying to patients, "Here's some clomiphene—take some each month and call me if you miss your period" should be deplored.

But if clomiphene citrate is taken under proper supervision and the woman has previously determined that she is not pregnant, its safety is beyond question. This has prompted many IVF programs to continue using it. Those that do so, however, invariably report a lower pregnancy rate than that which can be achieved by other methods of COH.

Letrozole: A New Oral Agent for Induction of Ovulation

Letrozole, like clomiphene, is an oral agent that induces ovulation. The main source of estrogen is through the conversion of the hormone testosterone to estrogen by the action of a follicular enzyme known as aromatase. Letrozole, an aromatase inhibitor, blocks this conversion, resulting in a reduction in the concentration of estrogen, which in turn causes the pituitary gland to release large amounts of FSH as well as LH. The FSH promotes follicle development. While the effect on pituitary FSH and LH release is similar to that of clomiphene, Letrozole does not block estrogen receptors in the endometrial lining or cervical glands and thus does not directly affect the production of cervical mucus (essential for sperm capacitation) or suppress development of the uterine lining.

However, as with clomiphene, Letrozole increases the release of LH. This, in turn, can lead to overproduction of male hormones (e.g., testosterone) by the ovaries with a potentially adverse effect on egg/embryo quality. This is potentially most disadvantageous in older women and women who have diminished ovarian reserve (i.e., raised FSH, reduced Inhibin B levels, and fewer than 10 antral follicles on cycle day 3) because their ovaries have the greatest potential of producing excessive testosterone.

Thus, while there could be potential advantages in using Letrozole over clomiphene for induction of ovulation, the exaggerated LH-induced testosterone effect, especially in women over 40 and/or those with evidence of diminished ovarian reserve, limits its value in the ART setting.

Gonadotropins (Urinary-Derived and Recombinant, Repronex, Bravelle, Follistim, Gonal F)

Urinary-derived gonadotropins, such as Repronex, contain equal amounts of FSH and LH, while the purified derivative, Bravelle, contains 98 percent FSH. These products are all derived from the urine of menopausal women, which is a good source of both FSH and LH. This is because a menopausal woman's pituitary gland, in response to a feedback message that her ovaries are no longer producing enough estrogen, increases the output of FSH and LH in an effort to restimulate the failing ovaries. The excess FSH and LH are excreted in the urine. Urine used for gonadotropins is distilled, filtered, and purified by an expensive process.

Too much of the LH component of gonadotropins directly stimulates the tissue surrounding the ovarian follicles, which propagates precursors that in turn produce *androgens* (male hormones). When present in excess in the ovaries, androgens may filter into the surrounding follicles and adversely affect both follicle and egg development. It is also possible that, in large concentrations, androgens such as testosterone would inhibit the proper development of the endometrial lining. In this way ovarian androgen production induced by LH could have a deleterious effect on egg and embryo quality as well as on the potential for healthy implantation in the endometrium. Accordingly, we have largely substituted purified FSH for urinary-derived gonadotropins products such as Repronex, which contain both FSH and LH, in most cases of ovarian stimulation in preparation for IVF. Finally, as with urinary-derived gonadotropin, variations in both interpersonal and intrapersonal responses due to the influence of isohormones are known to occur with purified FSH.

Today, most gonadotropins used in IVF are derived from "recombinant DNA technology" using genetic engineering (Follistim, Puregon, Gonal F).

At the time of the writing of this book, one vial of gonadotropins costs about $60 in the United States, and an IVF candidate could require 25 to 90 vials per treatment cycle, depending on her response.

If administered in sufficient amounts beginning early enough in the menstrual cycle, gonadotropins will prompt the development of a large number of follicles. Although the average number of eggs usually retrieved from a woman younger than 40 after gonadotropins stimulation—provided she has two ovaries—ranges between 10 and 15, retrievals of more than 50 eggs at one time have been reported.

Because gonadotropins cannot be absorbed through the stomach and intestinal walls into the bloodstream, they must be administered by injection rather than taken orally. The usual injection schedule is from day 2 or 3 through day 8 to 12 of the menstrual cycle.

One of the most significant attributes of gonadotropins is its safety-valve effect on ovulation. No matter how well stimulated a woman becomes when she takes gonadotropins, she will be unlikely to ovulate until she receives an injection of hCG. Thus, if for any reason it is determined that the woman should not progress to ovulation, the hCG is simply not administered.

Side effects of gonadotropins. Most women taking gonadotropins report breast tenderness, backaches, headaches, insomnia, bloating, and increased vaginal discharge, which are directly due to increased mucus production by the cervix.

Luteal-phase defects are also known to occur in association with gonadotropins therapy. However, endometrial biopsies have shown that the development of the uterine lining of patients stimulated with gonadotropins is usually a few days ahead of that which could be expected in unstimulated cycles. Thus, gonadotropins help to synchronize development of the endometrium with growth of the follicles and eggs. This synchronization is a critical prerequisite for successful implantation because IVF embryos are usually transferred to the uterus a few days earlier than they otherwise would reach it under natural circumstances. Therefore, accelerated endometrial development enhances the chances that the young embryos will implant after their transfer to the uterus.

Ovarian hyperstimulation syndrome (OHS). Women who undergo ovarian stimulation with gonadotropins and produce more than 25 follicles (of greater than 15 mm diameter) with a peak estradiol of more than 4000 pg/ml on the day of the hCG administration are at increased risk of developing severe *ovarian hyperstimulation syndrome* (OHS). Symptoms include some or all of the following: abdominal distention (due to fluid collection, i.e., *ascites*), rapid weight gain (of a pound or more a day), abdominal pain, lower backache, nausea, diarrhea, vomiting, spots in front of the eyes, and a declining urine output. These symptoms can start well before the first pregnancy test is performed; but if the woman fails to conceive, they will dissipate rapidly and spontaneously within two weeks thereof. If the woman conceives, however, the symptoms may become progressively worse. Either way, since this is a self-limiting condition that rapidly disappears after the eighth week of pregnancy, at which point ovarian support of the pregnancy is taken over by the placenta, the problem will almost always be gone by the 60th day of pregnancy (day 1 being the day that gonadotropins shots were initiated). Rapid resolution is usually heralded by frequent and extended visits to the bathroom to urinate as the fluid that collected in the abdomen rapidly passes out of the system.

Symptoms or signs of rapidly increasing abdominal fluid collection may become so severe as to compromise breathing or render the degree of discomfort intolerable. In such cases, most of the fluid should and can readily be drained by repeated (once or twice weekly) sterile vaginal needle aspiration (paracentesis) until the problem self-corrects at about the eighth week of pregnancy.

Urine output should be monitored daily to see if it drops below about 600ml a day (about two and a half cups). A chest X-ray to evaluate for fluid collection in the chest and around the heart should be done weekly along with blood tests for hematocryt, BUN, electrolytes, creatinine, platelet count, and fibrin degradation products (FDP). If indicated by a deteriorating situation, hospitalization might be needed for close observation and intensive care.

The ovaries will invariably be considerably enlarged in all cases of OHS. However, unless ovarian torsion (twisting of the ovary on its axis) occurs—and this is very rare indeed—ovarian enlargement is of little consequence.

OHS patients with ascites (fluid collection) are advised to raise the head of the bed slightly by placing a 4- to 6-inch block under each of the headposts and to use a few extra pillows to minimize ascitic fluid from splinting the diaphragm and making breathing difficult.

Since OHS is inevitably self-limiting, the idea is to try and prevent things from getting out of hand until it clears up on its own. Intervention should be confined to those cases where symptoms or signs point to rapid deterioration. It is important to know that symptoms are due to the effect of a rising hCG. Thus, feeling bad is often a "good sign," because symptoms that were to spontaneously disappear or fade prematurely could indicate that hCG levels were dropping, and this could mean that the pregnancy is in jeopardy.

Clearly, women with OHS should never receive additional hCG injections.

Prolonged coasting.   It has been demonstrated that if more than 25 follicles develop following stimulation with fertility drugs and the woman's blood estradiol at its highest level exceeds 6,000 pg/ml, there could be in excess of an 80 percent risk of the life-endangering complications described above.

Until relatively recently, the only way to prevent these complications from occurring was by withholding hCG in those cases where inadvertent overstimulation appeared to be taking place. In the mid-1990s, we introduced an approach that permits the cycle of treatment to continue while eliminating any significant risk of severe ovarian hyperstimulation. This new method can only be applied in cases where patients are being concurrently treated with *GnRHa* (gonadotropin-releasing hormone agonist). In cases where the advent of severe hyperstimulation is suspected, the gonadotropins therapy is withheld while the GnRHa treatment is continued, and the woman undergoes daily blood estradiol measurements until the concentration drops to a safe level. At that time hCG is administered, regardless of the number of developed follicles or the number of eggs retrieved; thus these women do not develop life-endangering complications. We term this method *prolonged coasting*. Prolonged coasting has essentially removed most of the major risks associated with the use of fertility drugs.

Precise timing of the initiation of prolonged coasting is critical. Reports of poor fertilization rates and poor embryo quality following use of this method are largely due to improper timing of the initiation of the coasting process.

Variations in response to gonadotropins.   Some women stimulate well after relatively small doses of gonadotropins. Others require two, three, or even four times that dosage to achieve the same effect. In the past, selecting the proper dosage was a trial-and-error process because there was simply no way to predict how a particular woman might respond. Each woman is unique, and each can be expected to react differently to gonadotropins. However, about 80 percent of women respond appropriately to an average injection.

We now measure FSH and blood estradiol on the second or third day of a natural menstrual cycle preceding the IVF cycle. We use the levels of these hormones to predict the probable way the woman will respond to a variety of stimulation methods. We believe these tests are also valuable in selecting the most appropriate dosage and regimen of fertility drugs to be administered.

Despite these refinements, however, stimulation for IVF is still something of a hit-or-miss procedure. For example, when a woman has used up most of her lifetime egg budget and is left with less than a critical number of eggs, she begins to enter a phase of hormonal change known as the *climacteric.* The climacteric is associated with a loss of fertility, the onset of hot flashes, and mood changes. It ultimately culminates with the total cessation of menstruation between the ages of 40 and 55, a process called *menopause.* The ovaries still produce hormones after menopause, but they are released in a constant rather than cyclical manner.

When a woman fails to become stimulated on the first try, hormone tests are indicated to ensure that she is not in the climacteric as well as to determine if hormonal abnormalities or other conditions might be inhibiting her sensitivity to gonadotropins. If she is not in the climacteric and no other abnormalities are detected, then it can be anticipated that she will eventually respond to an adjusted dosage of gonadotropins. She can begin another round of gonadotropins therapy with an adjusted dosage after she lets her body recover for a month or two.

Follicle growth and development, egg maturation, the number of eggs that can be retrieved, and the risk of side effects are directly related to the patient's response as evaluated by blood-estrogen levels and/or ultrasound, not to the dosage of gonadotropins. Therefore, it is illogical to fear administering an escalating dose of gonadotropins after a poor response to a standard dosage. What is important is to monitor the *individual's* response to the drug.

The tremendous interpersonal and intrapersonal variations in response to gonadotropins might be attributable to one or both of the following factors. It could be that hormonal and biochemical factors governing the response to gonadotropins vary in the different women or even at different stages of the same woman's life. For example, as we noted earlier in this chapter, age influences the woman's ovarian receptivity to gonadotropins, especially as she nears the climacteric. In addition, some women simply will not respond consistently to administration of the same dosage of gonadotropins from month to month.

Gonadotropin-Releasing Hormone Agonist (GnRHa)—Lupron, Synarel, Nafarelin, Buserelin

Drugs that inhibit the release of LH, called GnRH (gonadotropin-releasing hormone) agonists, or GnRHa, are now commonly used prior to or in combination with gonadotropins and FSH. This treatment reduces the number of canceled cycles by more than 60 percent. These drugs are marketed in the United States as Lupron, Synarel, Nafarelin, and Buserelin.

In about 25 percent of cases where women receive gonadotropins, a progressive increase in the production of LH, which eventually reaches a crescendo (the premature LH surge), leads to "follicular exhaustion," causing the follicle(s) to stop developing and damage the eggs. This results in a rapid fall in the blood estradiol concentration mandating cancellation of the treatment cycle. Moreover, studies show that many of the interpersonal variations in response to fertility drugs occur because some women release higher levels of LH into their blood than others. It was this finding that led to the suggestion that prevention of excessive exposure to LH in women being treated with fertility drugs could help standardize response to fertility agents. Some of these can be taken nasally as snuff or spray, or by daily injection.

One of the minor disadvantages of using GnRH agonists is that in some cases they can reduce the ovarian sensitivity to gonadotropins, thus requiring higher dosages of these drugs as well as their administration for a longer time than would otherwise have been necessary. However, the advantages of combining these two agents far outweigh the disadvantages.

The use of GnRH agonists represents a significant breakthrough in the treatment of infertility.

Gonadotropin-Releasing Hormone Antagonists (Cetrotide, Antagon, Cetrorelix)

Unlike GnRH agonists, which expunge most LH and FSH out of the pituitary, leading to their virtual disappearance from the blood as they are eliminated from the body over a number of days, GnRH antagonists work within hours to block the release of FSH and LH. As such, they have the following potential advantages over GnRH agonists: (1) GnRH antagonists evoke a rapid suppression of pituitary gonadotropins release; in fact, women who receive GnRH antagonists will have minimal blood levels of endogenous gonadotropins (FSH and LH produced by the pituitary gland) within 48 hours of the treatment being initiated; (2) GnRH antagonists reportedly do not competitively bind with ovarian FSH receptors and, accordingly, allow for a better response to stimulation by a given dosage of gonadotropins; and (3) the use of Antagon/Cetrotide allows for the initiation of COH to begin on short notice in the natural or oral contraceptive-treated cycle, thereby minimizing the need to postpone initiation of COH. (Oral contraceptives are often used to set up the cycle of stimulation.)

EVALUATION OF FOLLICULAR DEVELOPMENT

In order to properly schedule surgical retrieval of eggs, the IVF physician must be sure that proper follicular development has occurred.

Because IVF programs rely heavily on the woman's daily blood-estrogen levels and daily ultrasound measurements of follicular developments in order to fine-tune this scheduling, usually by day 9 to 14 of the cycle a go/no-go decision can be made about whether to proceed to egg retrieval.

The Role of Vaginal Ultrasound Evaluation

When undergoing an vaginal ultrasound examination, the woman can feel the pressure of the transducer in her vagina, but she cannot feel or hear the sound waves as they travel through body tissue and fluid, and form images on a TV-like screen. Ultrasound enables the physician to see the woman's ovaries clearly and to identify, count, and even measure the fluid-filled follicles as they develop, providing an important indicator of the expected time of ovulation.

The Importance of Measuring Blood Estradiol and Performing Ultrasound Follicular Assessments

Measurement of the level of the hormone estradiol in the blood gives an approximate indication of how many eggs the physician might expect to retrieve. In general, the higher the estradiol level, the more eggs. This test will usually be done daily during the latter part of the treatment cycle preceding egg retrieval. In some programs, the estradiol level is measured throughout the treatment cycle.

If a woman taking gonadotropins does not stimulate enough after a week or so, she can continue gonadotropins medication for a few more days while her response is monitored by blood tests and/or ultrasound examinations. Such a delay should not significantly decrease her chance of getting pregnant. In certain cases, a woman who has not received GnRH agonist will show an optimal response to gonadotropins followed by an unexpected drop in hormone levels prior to egg retrieval. This is usually an indication that the hormone LH has been spontaneously released prematurely, thus threatening the health of the follicles and eggs. When this occurs, the physician should cancel the treatment cycle, and should reassess both the method and dosage of stimulation in a subsequent cycle.

The Injection of hCG—A Safety Valve

When blood estradiol levels and/or ultrasound assessment indicate that the follicular development of a woman taking gonadotropins is enough to produce an adequate number of eggs but unlikely to cause dangerous side effects, she will be given an injection of hCG to ripen the follicles and eggs for ovulation. The hCG triggers ovulation, which occurs within 38 to 42 hours, in the same manner as does the surge of LH in nature.

Similar in structure to LH, hCG is favored for the induction of ovulation. (It is also the hormone measured to assess whether a woman is pregnant.) Because hCG is broken down and made inactive when it passes through the stomach if taken in pill form, it must be injected in order to be transported directly to the ovaries.

After the administration of hCG, egg retrieval is scheduled to be performed within about 36 hours (i.e., prior to the anticipated time of ovulation). The follicles will then continue to grow until the eggs are retrieved or ovulation occurs.

AN INDIVIDUALIZED APPROACH TO
INDUCTION OF OVULATION

In order for any organism to attain an optimal state of maturation it must first undergo full growth and development. A plum plucked from a tree before having developed fully, or a poorly developed plum, might still ripen (mature) on the windowsill, and might even look just as enticing, but the underdeveloped fruit will never achieve optimal quality. The same principles apply to the development and maturation of human eggs. Proper development as well as precise timing in the initiation of egg maturation with LH or hCG is no less crucial to optimal egg maturation, fertilization, and ultimately to embryo quality. In fact, in cases where egg maturation is improperly timed (LH or hCG is released/given too early or too late), there is an increased risk of structural and numerical chromosomal abnormalities leading to compromised reproductive performance.

The potential for a woman's eggs to undergo orderly development, maturation, successful fertilization, and subsequent progression to good-quality embryos capable of producing healthy offspring is, in large part, genetically determined. However, the expression of such potential is profoundly susceptible to numerous extrinsic influences, especially to intra-ovarian hormonal changes during the pre-ovulatory phase of the cycle.

During the normal ovulation cycle, ovarian hormonal changes are regulated to avoid irregularities in production and interaction that could adversely influence follicle development and egg quality. As an example, while small amounts of ovarian androgens, such as testosterone, enhance egg and follicle development, overexposure to excessive concentrations of the same hormones can seriously compromise egg quality. It follows that protocols for controlled ovarian hyperstimulation should be geared toward optimizing follicle and egg development while avoiding overexposure to androgens. The fulfillment of these objectives requires an individualized approach to COH and that the administration of hCG or LH to trigger ovulation be timed precisely.

It is important to recognize that LH and FSH, while both playing a pivotal role in follicle development, have different primary sites of action in the ovary. The action of FSH is mainly directed toward proliferation of the *granulosa cells*, which line the inside of the follicles, and estrogen production. LH, on the other hand, acts primarily on the *ovarian stroma*, the connective tissue that surrounds the follicles, to produce androgens. Only a small amount of testosterone is necessary for optimal estrogen production; overproduction has a deleterious effect on granulosa cell activity, follicle growth/development, egg maturation, fertilization potential, and, ultimately, embryo quality. Furthermore, excessive ovarian androgens can also compromise estrogen-induced endometrial growth and development.

In conditions such as *polycystic ovarian syndrome* (PCOS), which is often characterized by increased blood LH levels, there is also an increased ovarian androgen production. It is, therefore, not surprising

that poor egg/embryo quality and inadequate endometrial development are often features of this condition. The use of LH-containing
preparations such as Repronex further aggravates this effect. Thus, we
strongly recommend against the exclusive use of such drugs in PCOS
patients, preferring FSH-dominant products such as Follistim, Gonal F,
and Bravelle.

While it would seem prudent to limit LH exposure in *all* cases of
COH, this appears to be more relevant in women with PCOS, in those
with diminished ovarian reserve, and in older women, all of whom
tend to be more sensitive to LH.

It is common practice to administer GnRH agonists (e.g., Lupron,
Buserelin) and, more recently, GnRH antagonists (e.g., Antagon,
Cetrorelix, Cetrotide) to prevent the release of LH with COH (see
discussion of GnRH agonists and GnRH antagonists earlier in this
chapter).

Long GnRHa Protocols

The most commonly prescribed protocol for Lupron/gonadotropins
administration is the so-called long protocol. Lupron is administered
starting a week or so before menstruation in the cycle prior to the IVF
treatment cycle, and precipitates an initial rise in FSH and LH levels,
which is rapidly followed by a precipitous fall to near zero.
Menstruation then ensues, whereupon gonadotropins treatment is initiated to ensure a relatively LH-free environment while daily Lupron
injections continue.

Flare GnRHa Protocols

Another approach to COH is by way of so-called flare protocols. This
involves initiating gonadotropins therapy simultaneously with administration of GnRH agonist. The intent is to deliberately allow Lupron to
effect an initial surge ("flare") in FSH release in order to augment ovarian response to the gonadotropins medication. Unfortunately, this
approach is a double-edged sword, as the resulting increased release of
FSH is likely to be accompanied by a similar rise in blood LH levels that

could evoke excessive ovarian stromal androgen production. This could potentially compromise egg quality, especially in older women and in women with conditions like PCOS in which the ovaries have increased sensitivity to LH. We believe that in this way, flare protocols could potentially hinder endometrial development, compromise egg/embryo quality, and reduce IVF success rates. Accordingly, we prefer to avoid them.

GnRH Antagonist Protocols

The use of GnRH antagonists as currently prescribed in ovarian stimulation cycles may be problematic, especially in women with high LH and overgrowth (*hyperplasia*) of ovarian stroma (e.g., women over 40, women with raised cycle day 3 FSH and/or low Inhibin B, other poor responders to gonadotropins, and in some women with PCOS). In such cases, the initiation of pituitary suppression with GnRH antagonists *so late* in the cycle of stimulation fails to suppress relatively high tonic pituitary LH levels in the earliest stage of follicular growth and development. One of the roles of LH is to promote androgen production, which as previously stated, is essential *in small amounts* for optimal follicular growth to take place. In women with high LH and/or ovarian stromal hyperplasia, the failure of conventional GnRH antagonist protocols to address this issue results in the inevitable excessive exposure of follicles to androgens, mainly testosterone. This can adversely influence egg/embryo quality and endometrial development.

Presumably, the reason for the suggested mid-follicular initiation of high-dose GnRH antagonist is to prevent the occurrence of the so-called premature LH surge, which is known to be associated with "follicular exhaustion" and poor egg/embryo quality. However, the term *premature LH surge* is a misnomer, and the concept of this being a terminal event or an isolated insult is erroneous. In fact, the event is an end point in the progressive escalation in LH ("a staircase effect") with increasing ovarian stromal activation and commensurate growing androgen production. Trying to improve ovarian response so as to stave off follicular exhaustion by administering Antagon/Cetrotide during the final few days of ovarian stimulation is like trying to prevent a shipwreck through removing the tip of an iceberg. The use of such late-period follicular phase Antagon/Cerotide protocols in younger women or in normal responders will probably not produce such adverse effects because the tonic endogenous LH levels are low (normal) in such cases, and such normally ovulating women rarely have ovarian stromal hyperplasia. The better question would be: Do such women in fact require any form of pituitary suppression at all? We doubt that they do.

So, at SIRM we tend to favor prescribing 125 mcg Antagon or Cetrotide (i.e., half the usual dosage) starting on the day that FSH-dominant gonadotropins (Follistim, Gonal F, and Bravelle) stimulation is initiated, thus intentionally allowing a very small amount of the woman's own LH to enter her blood while preventing a large amount of LH from reaching her circulation. This is because while a small amount of LH is essential to promote and optimize FSH-induced follicular growth and egg maturation, a large concentration of LH can trigger overproduction of ovarian stromal testosterone with an adverse effect on follicle/egg/embryo quality. Moreover, since testosterone also down-regulates estrogen receptors in the endometrium, an excess of testosterone in the pelvic circulation can also have an adverse effect on endometrial growth.

Estrogen Priming Protocols

Older women (over 40 years), women who have demonstrated a prior reduced ovarian response to COH, and those who by way of significantly raised cycle day 3 FSH and reduced Inhibin B levels are considered likely to be poor responders and are first given GnRH agonist for a number of days to effect pituitary down-regulation. Upon menstruation and confirmation by ultrasound and blood estradiol measurement that adequate ovarian suppression has been achieved, the dosage of GnRH agonist is drastically lowered (or the agonist is replaced with a GnRH antagonist) and the woman is given twice-weekly injections of estradiol for a period of seven to ten days. COH is then initiated using a relatively high dosage of FSH-dominant gonadotropins (such as

Follistim or Gonal F) that is continued along with daily administration of GnRH agonist/antagonist until the hCG trigger is injected. A recently completed study has demonstrated the efficacy of this protocol and the ability to significantly improve ovarian response to gonadotropins in many hitherto resistant patients.

Agonist/Antagonist Conversion Protocols (A/ACP)

As alluded to above, the use of GnRH antagonists as currently prescribed in ovarian stimulation cycles (i.e., the administration of 250 mcg daily from the sixth or seventh day of stimulation with gonadotropins) may be problematic, especially in women with high LH and overgrowth (hyperplasia) of ovarian stroma (e.g., women over 40, women with raised cycle day 3 FSH and/or low Inhibin B, other "poor responders" to gonadotropins, and in some women with PCOS).

It is our position that some form of pituitary blockade, either in the form of a GnRH agonist or a GnRH antagonist is an essential component in ovarian stimulation of "poor responders" undergoing IVF. However, GnRH agonists have somewhat of a suppressing effect on ovarian response to gonadotropin stimulation. Thus, switching over from an agonist such as Lupron to an antagonist such as Antagon or Cetrotide at the onset of the Lupron-induced menstrual period (just prior to initiating ovarian stimulation with gonadotropins) may have significant benefits, especially in the treatment of "poor responders."

With the A/ACP, low-dose Antagon Cetrotide or Cetrorelix (125 mcg daily) is commenced at the onset of spontaneous menstruation or bleeding that follows initiation of GnRH agonist (e.g., Lupron) therapy using a long-down-regulation protocol arrangement and continuing until the day of the hCG trigger.

There is one potential drawback to the use of the A/ACP, in that the sustained use of a GnRH antagonist (e.g., Antagon/Cetrotide) throughout the stimulation phase of the cycle appears to compromise the predictive value of serial plasma estradiol measurements as a measure of follicle growth and development in that the estradiol levels tend to be much lower in comparison to cases where agonist (Lupron) alone is used or where a "conventional" GnRH antagonist protocol is employed (i.e., antagonist administration is commenced six to eight days following initiation of gonadotropin stimulation). Rather than being due to reduced production of estradiol by the ovary(ies), the lower blood concentration of estradiol seen with prolonged exposure to GnRH antagonist could be the result of a subtle, agonist-induced alteration in the configuration of the estradiol molecule, such that currently available commercial kits used to measure estradiol levels are rendered much less sensitive/specific. Thus when the A/ACP is employed, we rely much more heavily on ultrasound growth of follicles along with observation of the trend in the rise of estradiol levels than on absolute estradiol values. Thus we commonly refrain from prescribing the A/ACP in "high responders" who are predisposed to the development of severe ovarian hyperstimulation syndrome (OHSS) and accordingly where the accurate measurement of plasma estradiol plays a very important role in the safe management of their stimulation cycles.

It is remarkable that while using the A/ACP + E2V in "poor responders" whose FSH levels were often well above threshold limits, the cycle cancellation has consistently been maintained below 10 percent (i.e., much lower than expected). Many of these patients who had previously been told that they should give up on using their own eggs and switch to ovum donation because of "poor ovarian reserve" have subsequently achieved viable pregnancies at SIRM using the A/ACP with "estrogen priming."

We currently prescribe the A/ACP to most of our IVF patients regardless of whether they are "normal responders" or "poor responders." Preliminary results suggest a significant improvement in egg number and egg/embryo quality as well as in implantation and viable IVF pregnancy rates. The A/ACP has, however, proven to be most advantageous in "poor responders" where additional enhancement of ovarian response to gonadotropins may be achieved through incorporation of "estrogen priming." We have reported on the fact that the addition of estradiol for about a week following the initiation of the A/ACP, prior to commencing FSH-dominant gonadotropin stimulation, appears to further enhance ovarian response, presumably by up-regulating ovarian FSH-receptors. We refer to this as the A/ACP + E2V.

DOES THE USE OF GONADOTROPINS INCREASE THE RISK OF OVARIAN CANCER?

A paper that appeared in the medical literature about a decade ago suggested that the use of fertility agents might increase a woman's risk of subsequently developing ovarian cancer. The authors of this article, a group from Stanford University, computer analyzed data from 12 studies on ovarian-cancer patients done in the late 1970s and early 1980s. They compared data about ovarian-cancer patients with data about women of similar age and background who did not have the disease, looking for patterns relating to the incidence of ovarian cancer in infertile women who received fertility drugs.

In our opinion, this report made unsubstantiated and erroneous deductions for the following reasons. The only way to determine whether there is a link between fertility drugs and an increased occurrence of ovarian cancer would be through a prospective controlled study (a study in which data will be collected in the future) that compares two groups of infertile women: those who receive fertility drugs and those who do not.

Until the widespread introduction of IVF in the late 1980s, the reason most women were treated with fertility drugs such as clomiphene citrate and gonadotropins was because of abnormal or absent ovulation. More recently, due to the advent of assisted reproduction and intrauterine insemination, most women who receive fertility drugs ovulate normally; problems other than dysfunctional ovulation are at the root of their infertility.

Since the Stanford study reported on the use of fertility drugs prior to their widespread administration to normally ovulating women (for assisted reproduction), the study was biased. It would obviously take a very large controlled study to establish a definitive link between ovarian cancer and the use of fertility drugs. It is interesting that a few years ago the same journal that reported a link between ovarian cancer and the use of fertility drugs reported a follow-up on a large group of infertile women who received fertility drugs over a period of 12 years. This study failed to show any link with ovarian cancer.

Perhaps most important, the Stanford study did not adequately address the fact that because pregnancy has a protective effect against the development of ovarian cancer, those women who conceive through the use of fertility drugs might well have benefited from this treatment. The ultimate answer would come from a large prospective study aimed at evaluating the incidence of ovarian cancer in women who conceive following the use of fertility drugs versus those who fail to conceive in spite of such treatment. Such a study would take quite a long time to complete but would certainly identify the risk-benefit ratio associated with the use of fertility drugs.

We believe that the report suggesting an increased incidence of ovarian cancer with fertility drugs was poorly conceived, untimely, and inappropriate. It has added to the hurt of couples already ravaged by the emotional roller-coaster of infertility.

MOVING ON TO EGG RETRIEVAL

In summary, the woman who is optimally stimulated will, in our opinion, usually demonstrate a continuing rise or at least maintain a sustained level of blood estradiol while receiving gonadotropins. This would confirm that the follicles and eggs are continuing to develop optimally. It has been demonstrated that a large drop in the blood estradiol level after gonadotropins are discontinued is often associated with poor-quality eggs.

The optimum time for egg retrieval is about 34 to 36 hours after the final gonadotropins injection is administered.

The average number of eggs retrieved varies from program to program, depending on the patient population and the protocol of stimulation. We average between eight and 15 eggs per retrieval attempt (and can usually successfully fertilize about 70 to 80 percent of the mature eggs that we retrieve).

Overcoming the induction-of-ovulation hurdle is particularly significant in IVF. But in IVF, as in other important events in life, things don't always go as planned. Therefore, a reputable IVF program should counsel couples in preparation for the possibility that they may experience a poor stimulation cycle.

However, couples able to negotiate the induction-of-ovulation hurdle have a right to be guardedly optimistic about their overall chances of success. This is how one IVF physician encourages his patients and at the same time helps them maintain realistic expectations:

While the level of hormones and the ultrasound findings roughly correlate with the chances of retrieving a large number of eggs, this doesn't always hold true. Sometimes the follicles don't want to give up the eggs, or scar tissue may prevent us from reaching the ovary. And just because we retrieve an egg doesn't mean it will fertilize or that a fertilized egg will produce a "good-quality embryo." If we get a lot of eggs, that's great. I always emphasize that we have had many pregnancies result from the transfer of just one embryo.

6

IVF STEP 3:

EGG RETRIEVAL

Arrival at Step 3 represents a major accomplishment for IVF candidates because it means that the woman has been optimally prepared, both physically and emotionally, for egg retrieval. Now, for the first time in the treatment cycle, she and her partner have a realistic expectation of conceiving, because the IVF pregnancy rate is usually based on the chance of getting pregnant after undergoing egg retrieval. Their chance of success is now the pregnancy rate quoted by the program they have selected.

The egg retrieval phase exacts the greatest physical, emotional, and financial investment the couple will be expected to make in the entire treatment cycle. From egg retrieval onwards, the financial investment in IVF escalates sharply by the hour, largely because of the costs involved in the egg-retrieval procedure, laboratory fees for fertilization, and the embryo transfer. This outlay is particularly burdensome in the United States, where most couples must assume the entire expense since few insurance companies will fund these procedures.

THE PRE–EGG RETRIEVAL CONSULTATION

Prior to egg retrieval, the couple should have a refresher consultation with the physician who will actually perform the procedure. They should also meet with the rest of the IVF team that will be involved, including the nurses who will provide postoperative care.

The physician should explain the procedure in detail and describe how the woman might expect to feel afterwards. In addition, the physician should point out that although serious complications are highly unlikely, no one should undergo any kind of surgical procedure with the idea that it is devoid of risk. Although extremely rare, complications may include infection, bleeding, and injury to surrounding structures such as the bowel, bladder, or major blood vessels.

Because women who receive fertility drugs very often have corpus-luteum insufficiency, from the day of egg retrieval onwards many programs administer injections or vaginal suppositories containing progesterone to augment the production of progesterone by the corpus luteum. The physician who does so will probably discuss it with the couple at this point.

A consultation should also take place with the couple's anesthesiologist, who should review the woman's medical history, looking for conditions that could complicate the procedure. In the event that any such factors are detected, the anesthesiologist may call for an electrocardiogram, blood or urine tests, or other appropriate diagnostic measures in order to ensure that the surgery can proceed safely.

Finally, prior to the administration of any medication, the woman and her partner should be asked to decide what to do with the retrieved eggs and the embryos. The physician should reiterate the various scenarios previously discussed during the initial consultation, including a reminder that the more embryos transferred, the higher the pregnancy rate—with the concurrent risk of multiple pregnancy. The couple will usually be expected to issue a directive as to how many eggs they want fertilized, how many embryos (if any) should be frozen, and how many eggs or embryos (if any) may be donated. Finally, both partners will be asked to read and sign an informed-consent form that indicates they understand the egg-retrieval procedure and the risks associated with it.

ULTRASOUND-GUIDED EGG RETRIEVAL

Needle-aspirated egg retrieval under guidance by ultrasound can be performed in a doctor's office or in an outpatient surgery center environment.

Ultrasound-guided egg retrieval should be performed under conscious sedation and/or with the use of *paracervical block* for pain relief. A paracervical block is a procedure in which local anesthetic is injected on each side of the cervix to numb the nerves surrounding the uterus and cervix. At the same time, local anesthetic is also indicated into the upper part of the vagina surrounding the cervix. Some patients prefer to undergo the egg retrieval with the use of paracervical block alone, while the majority will prefer conscious sedation. (It is advisable than an anesthesiologist be present at the time of the egg retrieval.)

During ultrasound-guided egg retrieval, which almost always is done transvaginally, the physician will introduce a long ultrasound probe into the vagina. The probe is the projector that transmits the clearly identifiable image of each ovarian follicle to the ultrasound viewing monitor. The physician will then pass a sterile needle via a sleeve alongside the probe through the top of the woman's vagina into the ovarian follicles. The physician should be able to accurately direct the needle into the follicles by visualizing its progress on the ultrasound screen.

In the past, after the contents of the follicle were aspirated, the follicle was usually reinflated with a physiological solution in an attempt to flush out any egg that might otherwise have adhered to the wall of the follicle. Since this added a great deal of time to the procedure, it also created the necessity for prolonged conscious sedation. In addition, the injection of fluid through the aspiration needle would often reinject an egg lodged in the bore of the needle back into the follicle, making it far more difficult to aspirate a second time.

We believe that this flushing procedure is redundant in the vast majority of cases. Most important, it seldom improves the chances of harvesting more eggs. The rare exception might be in cases where the woman only has one or two follicles in her ovaries. Under such circumstances, the flushing process might ensure that the few eggs present will all be recovered.

Immediately following the procedure, the woman and her partner are informed as to the number and quality of eggs that have been retrieved. The egg retrieval procedure takes about 20 to 30 minutes, with approximately one hour of postoperative recovery. The woman can usually return to normal activity within a few hours of being discharged. The risk is negligible.

OBTAINING A SPECIMEN OF SEMEN TO FERTILIZE THE EGGS

The laboratory will need a semen specimen for insemination, which occurs four to six hours after egg retrieval. Although most men are able to produce a masturbation specimen upon demand, some may be unable to produce a specimen under the stress of the situation. If it is thought that this might happen, a backup specimen could be collected well in advance and frozen in liquid nitrogen or stored temporarily in special media.

The advantage of collecting a specimen a few days prior to egg retrieval is that the woman can assist her partner by creating circumstances in which he is more likely to be successful. In cases where obtaining a specimen by masturbation is difficult or inappropriate for religious or other reasons, the man can use a special condom while having intercourse so the specimen can be retrieved from the condom, or *coitus interruptus* can be performed.

In select cases it may be necessary to make a small hole at the end of the condom prior to intercourse and to collect the remaining sperm from the condom. The purpose of doing this is to make it possible for a small amount of sperm to pass from the condom into the vagina, thereby obviating religious objections by those sects that mandate that semen must reach the vagina for intercourse to be acceptable.

Although it has been suggested that thawed sperm usually fertilize eggs as well as a fresh specimen would, we have found that a fresh specimen is better, especially in cases of male infertility. We therefore recommend that even if the man has a frozen semen specimen available, he should attempt to produce a fresh specimen around the time when his partner's eggs are to be fertilized.

If the man has very poor sperm quality, it may be necessary for him to produce several daily specimens so they can be concentrated and frozen in case he cannot produce enough on the day of egg retrieval. In such cases it may also be advisable to enhance the quality of the sperm to improve their fertilizing capacity prior to capacitation in the IVF laboratory.

THE LABORATORY'S ROLE IN IVF

The IVF laboratory acts as a temporary womb that supports the delicate gametes and nurtures the newly formed embryos until they are transferred to the woman's uterus.

Nurturing the Eggs and Embryos

Even though the egg is the largest cell in the body, it is too small to be seen in the follicular flushings without a microscope. However, it is usually embedded in the collection of cells known as cumulus granulosa and collectively termed the corona radiata, which can be seen by the naked eye (see chapter 2). Once the corona radiata is identified in the follicular fluid, it is examined under the microscope to verify that it contains an egg. When the egg has reached optimal maturity it is placed in a petri dish in a nourishing liquid called an *insemination medium.* The insemination medium, which contains serum supplements, is a liquid environment that bathes and nourishes the eggs and embryos, just as in nature where the woman's body fluids nurture them in her reproductive tract. Each dish is carefully labeled with the couple's name, number, and perhaps even a colored label to guard against any mixup.

The insemination medium contains a common household product—baking soda, or sodium bicarbonate—which maintains the acid-alkaline balance (pH) of the medium at the same level as that found in the body. Without sodium bicarbonate the pH level would fluctuate because eggs and embryos, like any other living cells, convert oxygen, water, and food into waste products and excrete them into the surrounding environment. Sodium bicarbonate neutralizes these acidic and alkaline wastes so they do not threaten the well-being of the eggs and embryos.

Because sodium bicarbonate cannot perform this vital function without an adequate supply of carbon dioxide, the eggs and embryos are kept inside an incubator whose air supply contains a constant carbon-dioxide level of 5 percent. Under these conditions the sodium bicarbonate combines with the carbon dioxide to produce the chemical reaction that maintains the proper pH level in the insemination medium.

The embryos remain inside the incubator for the entire time they are in the laboratory, except for brief periods when they are temporarily removed in order to be microscopically examined and graded, changed to a new medium, or prepared for transfer to the uterus.

Sperm Washing and Capacitation

Freshly ejaculated sperm cannot fertilize an egg without undergoing capacitation. In the laboratory, sperm are washed in a special medium to induce capacitation before the insemination of the egg. As explained in chapter 2, capacitation involves altering the plasma membrane covering the acrosome on the sperm's head, thus releasing enzymes that will be needed for penetration and fertilization of the egg. Natural capacitation is performed by the fluids in the woman's reproductive tract, especially by the cervical mucus. In the laboratory, capacitation is accomplished by washing and then incubating the sperm at 37°C (body temperature) for about an hour.

The male partner's semen specimen can be prepared for insemination in a variety of ways. One way is to wash the semen in medium and process it in a centrifuge to separate the sperm from the seminal fluid. The sperm gravitate to the bottom of the container, and the seminal plasma is poured off and discarded. Additional medium is then added to the sperm, which are re-centrifuged until they again collect at the bottom of the container. At this point the used medium is discarded. New medium is added, and the washed sperm are placed in the incubator to complete the capacitation process.

Frequently, the sperm are allowed to swim through special columns of fluid that contain a substance called Percoll. The healthiest sperm can in this way be harvested from the bottom of such columns and used for insemination.

Caffeine-like substances are sometimes added to enhance sperm motility—to "wake them up," in effect. And incubation in follicular fluid obtained from one or more of the woman's follicles at the time of egg retrieval or in a special protein medium called *test yolk buffer* may improve the ability of the sperm to penetrate the egg.

Insemination

During *insemination,* the embryologist adds a drop or two of the medium containing capacitated sperm to the petri dish containing the egg(s). The egg, now surrounded by about 50,000 swimming sperm (the number contained in just two drops of fluid), is returned to the incubator and left undisturbed until the following morning. Fertilization, the actual entry of the sperm into the egg, normally occurs within the first few hours after insemination. In reputable laboratories, each harvested mature egg has a better than 70 percent chance of fertilization. However, if most or all of them fail to fertilize, one might suspect the existence of a previously undiagnosed fertility problem. This is an example of the dual role—both therapeutic and diagnostic—that IVF fulfills.

The Fertilized Egg

About 16 to 20 hours after insemination, the embryologist transfers each egg to a new growth medium in order to promote its development and encourage cell division if fertilization has occurred.

The most sophisticated IVF programs examine the eggs at this time to detect the presence of two nuclear bodies (one from the sperm and the other from the egg) within the egg itself. This *pronuclear* stage confirms that fertilization has actually taken place. It also enables the laboratory personnel to select embryos for cryopreservation at the most favorable time.

By now the corona radiata cells have condensed around the egg, obscuring its surface and preventing the embryologist from determining whether the egg has been fertilized. In nature, the cumulus granulosa and corona radiata cells are eroded away as the fertilized egg, or zygote, as it is called now, passes through the fallopian tube on its way to the uterus. In the laboratory, these cells must be skillfully removed, or "peeled," to avoid damaging the delicate embryo. Peeling is achieved by sucking the zygote and its attached corona into a small-gauge syringe needle or a fine-bore glass pipette and then flushing the zygote out through the narrow opening, thus separating it from the corona.

If more than two pronuclei (conglomerates of chromosomal material, *polyploidy*) are present, the fertilized egg will not produce a viable embryo. Because it was previously erroneously believed that the presence of more than two pronuclei was due to fertilization of the egg by more than one sperm, the condition was in the past inaccurately termed "polyspermia." The better term is *polyploidy*. Polyploidic eggs are discarded because they do not have the potential to grow into a baby. In some cases, however, it is not possible to diagnose polyploidy because in order to do so, the fertilized egg must be visualized very early on in its developmental process. In such cases, one or more polyspermic embryos might be inadvertently transferred into the woman's uterus. However, this does not cause a major risk to the woman because the polyspermic embryo, like most abnormal embryos, is highly unlikely to implant.

Over the last decade, many IVF labs have taken to adding cells derived from the growth of other tissue (from the lining of follicles, the fallopian tubes, Vero cells, etc.) to the culture medium in which the zygote is being nurtured ("co-culturing of the embryos"). It was initially believed that this technique added valuable cell-derived growth-promoting factors to the medium and that they might even in some way direct the embryo to develop in a healthier manner. However, the absence of convincing evidence that embryo co-culturing affords a real benefit has led to a decline in the popularity of this technique.

The zygote will not begin to divide for several more hours; once it divides, it is known as an embryo. The process of cell division is called *cleavage.*

About 46 hours after egg retrieval, the embryo is examined under a microscope. By now the cleaved embryo is a translucent, amber-colored mass of two to six cells (blastomeres). At this time, we transfer the embryos into blastocyst media. Within 72 hours of insemination most healthy embryos will have divided into seven to nine blastomeres.

Slower-dividing embryos (i.e., those that are less than seven blastomeres at 72 hours post-insemination) are much less likely to produce viable pregnancies. Similarly, embryos of greater than nine blastomeres as well as those that within 72 hours of insemination have already begun compacting their blastomeres together are also less likely to produce viable pregnancies. By 96 hours the healthy embryo will have more than 80 blastomeres and will look like a mulberry, or morula. By 120 to 144 hours after insemination, most viable embryos will comprise more than 100 cells and have a fluid-filled center or blastula, and are said to be at the blastocyst stage. Once transferred to the uterus, the viable embryo or blastocyst "hatches" from the zona pellucida and begins to implant into the uterine lining within 24 to 48 hours.

Figure 6-1 is a flow chart that summarizes the conventional IVF process in the laboratory from egg retrieval to embryo transfer.

INTRACYTOPLASMIC SPERM INJECTION (ICSI)

The procedure of *intracytoplasmic sperm injection (ICSI)* involves the direct injection of a single sperm into each egg under microscopic vision. The successful performance of ICSI requires a high level of technical expertise. In centers of excellence, when ICSI is employed the IVF birthrate is unaffected by the presence and severity of male infertility. When there is an absence of sperm in the ejaculate such as occurs in cases of congenital absence of the major sperm-collecting ducts (vasa deferentia), following vasectomy, and in some cases of testicular failure or where the man has no sperm in the ejaculate, ICSI can be performed with sperm obtained through testicular sperm extraction (TESE) or testicular sperm aspiration (TESA), procedures in which sperm is removed directly from the testicles. With the exception of testicular failure, the birthrate is usually no different from when IVF is performed for indications other than male infertility, in such cases.

The introduction of ICSI has made it possible to fertilize eggs with sperm derived from men with the severest degrees of male infertility and in the process to achieve pregnancy rates as high if not higher than those which can be achieved through conventional IVF performed in cases of non-male-factor infertility.

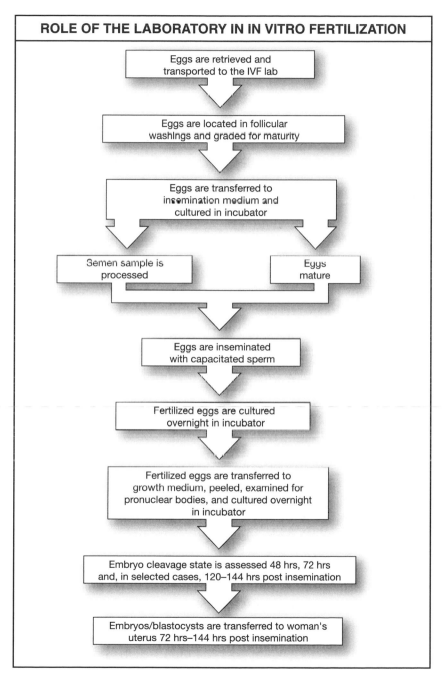

ROLE OF THE LABORATORY IN IN VITRO FERTILIZATION

Eggs are retrieved and transported to the IVF lab

Eggs are located in follicular washings and graded for maturity

Eggs are transferred to insemination medium and cultured in incubator

Semen sample is processed

Eggs mature

Eggs are inseminated with capacitated sperm

Fertilized eggs are cultured overnight in incubator

Fertilized eggs are transferred to growth medium, peeled, examined for pronuclear bodies, and cultured overnight in incubator

Embryo cleavage state is assessed 48 hrs, 72 hrs and, in selected cases, 120–144 hrs post insemination

Embryos/blastocysts are transferred to woman's uterus 72 hrs–144 hrs post insemination

FIGURE 6-1

The indications for ICSI have broadened dramatically, with the process now being used for a variety of indications other than male-factor infertility. For example, ICSI is often used to assist in the fertilization of eggs that are believed to have a hardened or thickened zona pellucida. This is frequently found in association with PCOS and in eggs derived from women over 40. ICSI is also frequently recommended in cases of unexplained infertility and where there is a history of poor fertilization during one or more prior IVF attempts.

As a consequence of ICSI, the treatment of male-factor infertility has emerged as one of the true success stories in the field of reproductive medicine.

Should ICSI Be Recommended in All Cases?

The performance of ICSI in cases of male-factor infertility has indeed been shown to slightly increase the risk of certain embryo chromosome deletions in the resulting embryos leading to an increase in early miscarriages. Also, male offspring resulting from ICSI-derived embryos could be at increased risk of being infertile in later life. However, it is important to stress that there is no evidence of a real increase in the incidence of serious birth defects attributable to the ICSI procedure itself. In fact, when ICSI is performed for indications *other than* male infertility, there is *no* reported increase in the risk of subsequent embryo chromosome deletions, miscarriages, or subsequent male-factor infertility in the offspring. But most importantly, given these drawbacks there is no alternative to ICSI in male infertility.

Because 12 to 15 percent of conventional IVF procedures are negatively affected by unanticipated absent or poor fertilization, some people have concluded that male infertility may be an "occult phenomenon" in some men. New tests of sperm DNA integrity (SDI) have demonstrated that DNA damage may be present in sperm from men with both normal and abnormal semen analyses, and that male infertility is equally prevalent in such cases. Thus, disappointments associated with unanticipated failed fertilization might be averted through routine performance of ICSI. There simply does not seem to be any practical downside to ICSI, and it is now routine throughout the SIRM system.

Another major advantage of conventional ICSI is that it affords the opportunity to remove the cumulus complex of cells that envelop the harvested egg and so enable the embryologist to evaluate microscopic parameters that point to maturity. This cannot be done with conventional IVF as the removal of these cells would virtually preclude conventional fertilization in the petri dish.

EMBRYO/BLASTOCYST CRYOPRESERVATION

When deciding what to do with the embryos in excess of those that will be transferred to the uterus, the couple undergoing IVF may have chosen cryopreservation.

Available evidence suggests that the transfer of thawed embryos/ blastocysts into the uterus does not increase the risk of birth defects. In addition, there have been dramatic advances in the technology of freezing and storing human embryos that hold great promise for the infertile couple.

At SIRM, with some exceptions, we prefer to cryopreserve embryos at 120 to 144 hours, as blastocysts, depending upon the couple's preference. Regardless of when the freezing process is done, we usually transfer embryos to the uterus at the blastocyst stage. This means that earlier embryos are thawed and cultured for a few days to develop further. Those that attain the blastocyst stage are eligible for transfer. Frozen blastocysts are thawed and then transferred a few hours later.

Approximately 10–15 percent of frozen blastocysts will likely be lost during the freeze-thaw process. However, recent technological advances have enhanced embryo/blastocyst freeze-thaw survival rates, resulting in a significant improvement in pregnancy rates following *frozen embryo transfer* (FET).

We believe that cryopreservation technology will continue to advance rapidly and will contribute significantly to the treatment of infertility in general and to successful IVF in particular. However, the future lies in the successful cryopreservation of human eggs (see chapter 15). While there has been definite progress in this arena, the poor egg freeze-thaw survival rate still precludes the widespread application of this technology in the clinical area.

7

IVF STEP 4:

EMBRYO TRANSFER

Although embryo transfer is the shortest step in an IVF procedure and appears at first glance to be the simplest, it is really the most critical phase of the entire process. Successful clearance of the previous hurdles means nothing if there is a bad transfer with bleeding, pain, and/or damage to the embryos. These problems can occur if too much time elapses between removal of the embryos from the incubator and their transfer into the uterus. A problem-free embryo transfer is so important that we even grade transfers in our setting on the basis of comfort, technical difficulty, and elapsed time so the staff can gauge its success. (In this chapter the term *embryo transfer* also refers to the transfer of blastocysts.)

Most embryo transfers are performed 72 to 144 hours after insemination or ICSI, but the actual time may depend on the state of cleavage of the most rapidly dividing embryo(s). Most programs prefer to perform embryo transfer before the leading embryo has advanced beyond the eight-cell stage; however, not all the embryos will be at the same stage of division when they are transferred, because they develop at different rates.

THE PRE-TRANSFER CONSULTATION

The couple's first step on the day of embryo transfer is a conference with the embryologist and the physician, with or without the clinical coordinator. The discussion will include the number and quality of the embryos and their cleavage state. The couple will already have discussed with the physician the optimal number of embryos that should be transferred to the uterus, given the woman's age. Some vacillation over what to do with all the embryos is to be expected up to this point, but now it is time for the couple to come to terms with the success rate vs. a high-order multiple pregnancy trade-off, as well as with the disposition of any remaining embryos.

The physician should describe what the couple can expect during the procedure (details vary widely from clinic to clinic). Some programs, particularly those located in hospitals, perform the embryo transfer in an operating room or a special procedure room, after which the woman is wheeled out on a gurney to a holding area until she has been discharged. Other programs prefer to perform the embryo transfer in the room where the woman will remain for an hour or two.

Some IVF programs allow the woman's partner to observe the transfer, while others require that he or she wait in another room. In some settings the couple cannot be together until the woman goes home, even if she has to relax for several hours after the transfer. Other programs, including our own, encourage the couple to be together during and after embryo transfer. We believe this facilitates the bonding process.

The physician should explain that the embryos are transferred with a thin catheter threaded through the cervix into the uterus. In programs such as ours, where the depth of the woman's uterus has been determined some days prior to the embryo transfer, the woman should be told that the embryos will be transferred to a specific depth just short of the top of the uterus to avoid injuring the endometrium. The intent here is to avoid any injury that might cause bleeding, which has a detrimental effect on the uterus.

THE EMBRYO TRANSFER

Undoubtedly, embryo transfer is the single most important step in IVF. It takes confidence, dexterity, and skill to perform a good transfer. Of all the procedures in ART, embryo transfer is the most difficult to teach.

Many women fail to conceive simply because the practicing physician could not perform this procedure optimally.

Shortly before the transfer, the embryos are put in a single petri dish containing growth medium. The laboratory staff then informs the clinical coordinator that the embryos are ready for transfer, and the coordinator prepares the patient and informs the physician that a transfer is imminent.

Ultrasound-Guided Embryo Transfer—A Must

Today all embryo transfers should be performed under direct ultrasound guidance to ensure proper placement in the uterine cavity. This practice, properly conducted, will significantly enhance embryo implantation and pregnancy rates.

We prefer to perform all embryo transfers when the woman has a full bladder. This facilitates visualization of the uterus by abdominal ultrasound and triggers a reflex nerve response that relaxes the wall of the uterus, reducing the likelihood of contractions occurring that could expel the embryo(s). The patient is allowed to empty her bladder 15 minutes following the embryo transfer.

It is important that the woman be as relaxed as possible during the embryo transfer because many of the hormones that are released during times of stress, such as adrenaline, can cause the uterus to contract. Accordingly, we offer the woman undergoing IVF in our program 5 mg of oral diazepam (Valium) about a half hour prior to the embryo transfer to relax her and reduce apprehension. Some IVF programs believe that imagery helps the woman relax and feel positive about the experience, thereby reducing the stress level. In such a program a counselor and/or clinical coordinator may help the woman focus on visual imagery for a few minutes immediately prior to embryo transfer so as to enhance her relaxation. As one clinical coordinator explained, couples may select a variety of creative images to visualize during embryo transfer:

I encourage them to visualize the uterus and the embryo growing within it. Some people imagine little embryos with suction cups on their feet—one woman imagined embryos with Velcro-covered feet. Some like to visualize a white light coating the baby or a peaceful blue halo surrounding the embryo, or a baby blanket giving the baby a hug, or little soldiers marching into the uterus and digging foxholes in the endometrium. No matter what our counselor or I suggest, the best visualization is what the woman thinks up for herself.

And I'm continually amazed at some of the lucky charms people bring along to the transfer. I have seen them bring drawings and paintings of babies. Some patients wear fertility charms, such as frogs or African face-mask pendants. Some listen to positive-reinforcement tapes. Women have told me they had worn their lucky dress—and I must confess that sometimes I've worn my lucky dress, too. You can't help getting caught up in this process.

When the woman is sufficiently relaxed, she is helped into the appropriate position and made as comfortable as possible. (In programs that rely on relaxation therapy, a counselor or nurse is usually present at the woman's bedside, coaching her in relaxation exercises during the procedure.)

The physician first inserts a speculum into the vagina to expose the cervix and then may clean the cervix with a solution to remove any mucus or other secretions. An abdominal ultrasound transducer is placed on the lower abdomen, and the uterus is clearly visualized. The physician then informs the embryology laboratory that the transfer is imminent and awaits the arrival of the transfer catheter loaded with the embryos.

The physician gently introduces the catheter through the woman's cervix into the uterine cavity under ultrasound guidance. When the catheter is in place, the embryologist carefully injects the embryos into the uterus, and the physician slowly withdraws the catheter. The catheter is immediately returned to the laboratory, where it is examined under the microscope to make sure that all the embryos have been deposited. Any residual embryos would be re-incubated, and the transfer process would usually be repeated to deliver the remaining embryos.

An embryo-transfer procedure usually takes only a few minutes from start to finish, although it naturally takes longer if the embryos must be re-incubated prior to a second or third transfer attempt.

In rare situations where a previously performed mock embryo transfer (a probe or a embryo-transfer catheter has been introduced via the cervix into the uterine cavity to determine the exact depth of the uterus) revealed that it would be impossible to pass the catheter through the cervix, the physician might then elect to perform a *transmyometrial embryo transfer* to the uterus. In this procedure, with the patient under general anesthesia, the physician, using a vaginal ultrasound probe, introduces a relatively wide-bore needle transvaginally through the wall of the uterus into the uterine cavity. The catheter containing the embryos is passed through this needle into the uterus, the embryos are delivered into the uterine cavity, and the needle and catheter are withdrawn.

After the Transfer

The woman's partner or another companion is expected to remain with her for emotional support and otherwise tend to her needs for the one hour she remains recumbent.

What the woman should expect to experience physically after embryo transfer is another important issue the physician would have discussed with the couple so they do not become unnecessarily concerned that the transfer has failed. For example, it is not unusual for the woman to experience minor lower-abdominal pain or a slight discharge after the transfer. This discharge may merely be due to the emission of fluid retained in the vagina as a consequence of cleaning the cervix in preparation for embryo transfer.

THE EXIT INTERVIEW

The exit procedure varies from program to program, but every couple is entitled to an exit interview prior to leaving the IVF clinic. An exit interview prepares and reassures couples for their return home and also provides valuable feedback to the IVF program. During the exit interview, the couple and the physician and/or clinical coordinator discuss follow-up care, including permissible daily activity, work, travel, and when the couple can resume sexual intercourse. The woman would be advised at this time whether the program recommends hormone supplementation until the pregnancy test confirms or rules out successful IVF. Some programs telephone patients after they have returned home to inquire about their emotional stability and physical well-being. The staff of such programs would likely emphasize that whether or not the procedure has been successful, they would still like to maintain contact with the couple and would be available for consultation at all times.

FOLLOW-UP AFTER THE EMBRYO TRANSFER

The Quantitative Beta hCG Blood Pregnancy Test

About 11 days after the egg retrieval, the woman should have a quantitative Beta hCG blood pregnancy test, which can diagnose pregnancy even before she has missed a period. It does so by determining the presence of the hormone hCG, which is produced in minute amounts by the implanting embryo. If hCG is detected, the test is usually repeated two days later in order to see if there has been an appreciable rise in hCG since the first test. (We usually recommend that these blood samples be drawn 11 and 13 days following the egg retrieval.) A doubling of the initial value usually suggests that an embryo is implanting and is a good indication of a possible pregnancy. The laboratory then notifies the IVF clinic of the test results.

Because an IVF program usually cooperates closely with the referring physician, it is customary for the clinic staff to call the referring physician with the results of the pregnancy test and ask the physician to notify the couple. Thereupon, the clinic staff may also contact the couple. Obviously, if the couple had selected the clinic themselves rather than on referral, the staff would call them directly with the test results.

Sometimes the physician or clinical coordinator will work through the referring physician to arrange for the pregnancy tests, and the program may also forward a detailed report about the entire procedure to the referring physician. If the couple wishes to make their own arrangements, the program should give them detailed instructions about the necessary tests.

Hormonal Support of a Possible Pregnancy

If the two blood-pregnancy tests indicate that one or more embryos are implanting, some programs advocate daily injections of progesterone or the use of vaginal hormone suppositories for several weeks to support the implanting embryo(s). Others give hCG injections three times a week for several weeks until the pregnancy can be identified by ultrasound. Some IVF programs do not prescribe any hormones at all after the transfer.

Progesterone vs. hCG Supplementation

This is by no means a clear-cut issue. Just as ovulation occurs following the spontaneous LH surge and/or the administration of gonadotropins following COH, resulting in a corpus luteum that produces both progesterone and estrogen, a similar but exaggerated response follows IVF, where COH with hCG-induced ovulation results in the formation of numerous corpus lutea. The greater the original number of mature follicles, the greater the progesterone/estrogen production is likely to be. Since ovarian stimulation in women who have abnormal or no ovulation patterns at all (e.g., cases of PCOS) tends to result in the growth of many more follicles than when performed in normally ovulating women, it follows that such women also tend to develop many more corpora lutea and accordingly have exaggerated progesterone/estrogen blood concentrations.

The hCG injection following embryo transfer exerts a protracted influence on ovarian progesterone/estrogen production that is sustained for at least one week. A few days later, provided that embryo implantation takes place, the early *trophoblast* (root system of the conceptus, which subsequently develops into the placenta) begins to produce its own progesterone/estrogen, as well as hCG, in ever-increasing amounts.

There is compelling evidence to show that hCG promotes the release of corpus luteum progesterone following ovulation as well as trophoblastic growth and development following embryo transfer; therefore, hCG enhances both progesterone and estrogen production while simultaneously promoting further hCG as well as progesterone/estrogen production by the trophoblast. As such, hCG might be considered a self-propagating hormone.

When hCG is administered following embryo transfer, the dosage is 5000 units by injection three times weekly beginning after early biochemical confirmation that implantation is taking place; hCG (whether self-produced or administered by injection) enhances the propagation and release of both ovarian and trophoblastic progesterone, which promotes further development of the uterine endometrial lining, trophoblastic growth, uterine relaxation, and adaptation of the reproductive immune response.

The trophoblast produces progesterone/estrogen in ever-increasing amounts so that by the eighth to ninth week of pregnancy it replaces the ovaries as the dominant source of production. Thus, there is probably little benefit through either hCG or progesterone administration after the completion of the 10th week of pregnancy. It follows that a low progesterone blood level is much more likely to be the consequence rather than cause of a failing pregnancy. This is the reason why many authorities believe that progesterone supplementation in such cases will not rescue a failing pregnancy.

Even the most adamant supporters of hCG supplementation recognize that its administration in some cases could bear risk. One such example is when, following COH with gonadotropins, the woman inadvertently becomes severely hyper-stimulated, placing her at risk of developing life-endangering complications associated with severe ovarian hyperstimulation syndrome (OHSS). In such cases, the administration of additional hCG often exacerbates the condition, thus increasing risk. We would prefer to administer progesterone in such cases although it is questionable whether there is any clinical benefit in doing so. A situation where progesterone rather than hCG clearly should be given is where the woman is an embryo recipient (e.g., ovum donation, embryo adoption, gestational surrogacy, or frozen-embryo transfer). In such cases, ovarian hormonal activity is dormant, and any attempt to promote progesterone/estrogen production would be fruitless.

Once reliance upon the corpus luteum to sustain the pregnancy completely transforms into total self-maintenance of the pregnancy by the placental trophoblast, supplementation with either progesterone or hCG is probably of limited, if any, benefit to the maintenance of the pregnancy. This is why after the completion of the eighth week of pregnancy, supplemental hormonal therapy is slowly tailed off and stopped altogether.

Women undergoing third-party parenting through IVF surrogacy or ovum donation will usually receive estrogen and progesterone injections, often in conjunction with vaginal hormone suppositories, for eight to ten weeks following the diagnosis of implantation by blood-pregnancy testing.

We believe it could, in special circumstances, be beneficial to administer hCG prior to performing the Beta hCG test for pregnancy diagnosis in order to provide better support for the possible pregnancy. This has been practiced selectively in our setting as well as in other IVF programs, and the results are encouraging. The problem with this approach is that administration of hCG prior to the test delays the ability to diagnose pregnancy because hCG is the very hormone that is measured to see if the woman is pregnant.

Confirming a Pregnancy by Ultrasound

Although a positive Beta hCG blood-pregnancy test indicates the possibility of a conception, pregnancy cannot be confirmed until it can be defined by ultrasound (see chapter 11 for a discussion of the various definitions of pregnancy). Three to four weeks after embryo transfer, ultrasound can confirm that a pregnancy exists, that it is viable through detection of a heartbeat, and that it is not ectopic.

What to Do If Spotting Occurs

The woman may experience a minimal degree of spotting (vaginal bleeding) after IVF, whether or not she is pregnant. If spotting occurs, she should call her physician immediately and rest in bed. Spotting can be caused by a variety of factors: (1) One of the embryos could be burrowing into the endometrium, (2) one could be attaching while another is detaching, (3) the menstrual period may have begun, or (4) the woman may have an ectopic pregnancy. Although there is no way of knowing in the very early stages exactly what is causing the spotting, certain tests can help isolate the problem.

Some women who spot after a positive pregnancy test are undergoing a spontaneous reduction of a multiple pregnancy. For example, many IVF as well as natural pregnancies start off as twins or even triplets and then spontaneously reduce themselves to a singleton or twin pregnancy. Painless bleeding might occur in the process, which could be falsely construed as an indication that the pregnancy is about to be lost.

All women should take the Beta hCG pregnancy test after IVF no matter how much they bleed. As one nurse-practitioner explained:

We had one patient who took her first pregnancy test, but since it was low she didn't take the second one. She kept spotting and spotting, and then went back to her aerobics—three hours every day. After about four weeks I called her up and asked how things were going. She said she had never really had her period and was having these pregnancy symptoms. . . . It turned out that she had conceived in spite of everything!

Women who do not get pregnant and want to make another attempt at IVF should wait until they have had at least one full unstimulated menstrual cycle in order to prepare themselves emotionally and give their ovaries a rest before the next procedure.

When an IVF pregnancy has been confirmed by symptoms and by ultrasound examinations, the woman should seek prenatal care as soon as possible. Thereafter, an IVF pregnancy can be expected to progress no differently from any normally conceived pregnancy given the woman's health, age, and related conditions.

8

THE FIVE ULTIMATUMS FOR SUCCESSFUL IVF CANDIDATES

Years ago, if a woman was pregnant over the age of 35, she was often placed at high risk for childbirth. Not only was it almost unthinkable that a woman over 40 would have a baby, it was strongly discouraged. Now many women in their forties and even in their fifties are having babies, often through the use of donated eggs. The point to be emphasized is that in order to get good success rates with IVF, it is important to eliminate as many as possible of the variables that might impact adversely on outcome before actually undertaking the IVF process itself. This chapter discusses these variables—which we refer to as "The Five Ultimatums":

1. Quality of the Woman's Eggs: The First Ultimatum
2. Quality of the Man's Sperm: The Second Ultimatum
3. Quality of the Embryo: The Third Ultimatum
4. Receptivity of the Uterus: The Fourth Ultimatum
5. Quality of the Embryo Transfer: The Fifth Ultimatum

In this chapter we will describe these ultimatums and explain how they may impact a couple's fertility. In chapter 9 we will describe the diseases that can impact infertility and in chapter 10 we will discuss tests that might be administered to both partners to determine the scope of their infertility. Chapter 10 suggests how a couple can use this knowledge to help determine what they can reasonably expect from IVF.

QUALITY OF THE WOMAN'S EGGS: THE FIRST ULTIMATUM

The Influence of Age on Egg Quality

Age is one of the most powerful variables to impact the five ultimatums, as well as other factors leading to a successful pregnancy. In fact, all forms of ART, including IVF, are associated with a reduced pregnancy rate in women over 40. Moreover, the cost of treatment is likely to be greater for older women because they often require more IVF cycles before there is likely to be a successful outcome. Infertile couples in which the woman is 40 or over must often overcome two hurdles when they seek fertility treatment: (1) desperation brought about by the realization that time is running out and (2) IVF programs that turn away women over a certain age. Advancing age associated with a progressive decline in a woman's natural fertility understandably induces an overwhelming sense of urgency to achieve a healthy pregnancy before time runs out. Less reasonable is the practice by some programs of turning away older women because their anticipated lower pregnancy rates could decrease the program's overall statistics so dramatically. Fertility drugs might only help a woman produce a greater number of eggs, not necessarily improve their quality. Thus, egg quality is a limiting parameter that must be met if the woman is to conceive. However, we do not believe in assigning arbitrary limits, such as an age-cutoff point beyond which we will not accept IVF candidates. We believe it is far more effective to enable each woman to estimate the probability of conceiving based on how the factors that impact fertility apply to her.

After the very onset of a woman's menstruation (i.e., the *menarche*), eggs are used up monthly until the number remaining in the woman's ovaries falls below a certain critical threshold, at which time ovarian function starts to decline and the woman becomes relatively resistant to ovarian stimulation with fertility drugs. This phase of the woman's reproductive life, the climacteric, is heralded by gradually increasing blood concentrations of FSH and a decline in Inhibin B levels. The climacteric continues for six to eight years until virtually all remaining eggs have been used up, at which time ovulation and menstruation cease altogether, and the woman has reached menopause.

The timing of the onset of the climacteric varies from person to person. Genetic factors, exposure to environmental toxins and radiation, disease, drugs, and pelvic disease associated with severe peri-ovarian adhesions that compromise blood flow to the ovaries can all influence timing of the onset of both the climacteric and menopause. Most American women will enter the climacteric in their early to mid-40s and go into menopause around ages 45 to 52.

Reduced egg quality is directly related to the woman's age. In contrast, reduced ovarian response to fertility drugs results from progressively declining ovarian function. As a woman advances beyond 30, each mature egg becomes progressively less likely to be "normal." In other words, with every advancing year fertilization is more likely to produce embryos that have an abnormal chromosome number (*aneuploidy*). At age 35 approximately one in three embryos is likely to be aneuploidic, while at 40 aneuploidy affects about 60 percent of the embryos. At age 42 approximately 70 percent of embryos are so affected, and at 45 the incidence of aneuploidy could be as high as 85 percent. Interestingly, 90 percent of embryo aneuploidy stems from chromosomal abnormalities originating in the egg rather than the sperm.

Since it is nature's intent to protect the integrity of the species through natural selection, abnormal embryos usually will fail to implant into the uterine lining or will be rejected in the first three months of pregnancy as a miscarriage. (In the case of failed implantation, the woman would probably not even be aware that she was actually pregnant for a very brief time). Infrequently, nature will make a mistake and allow a chromosomally defective fetus to continue on to delivery, resulting in conditions such as Down syndrome (Trisomy 21).

The negative effect of advancing age on egg quality not only explains why there is a gradual increase in the incidence of infertility, miscarriage, and chromosomal birth defects, it also illustrates why treatment of infertility, regardless of the chosen method, becomes progressively less successful with advancing maternal age.

Since onset of the climacteric usually (but not always) occurs when the woman is over 40, many physicians erroneously attribute poor egg quality to a reduction of ovarian responsivity to fertility drugs. However, a woman over 40 who has entered the climacteric would not only be far more likely to produce fewer eggs even following the administration of relatively high doses of fertility drugs, but because of her age a higher percentage of her eggs are likely to be chromosomally abnormal. Accordingly, her chances of having a baby using her own eggs would be reduced. Conversely, a woman over 40 undergoing IVF who has not yet entered the climacteric might yield many more eggs, thereby increasing the opportunity to select more and better-quality embryos for transfer.

It is the embryo quality rather than simply the number of embryos transferred to the uterus that influences the incidence of multiple pregnancies. Thus, the further the woman has advanced beyond 40, the less likely she will be able to have a multiple pregnancy even following the transfer of relatively large numbers of embryos. Therefore, the only way to optimize IVF birthrates in older women is to select the best-quality embryos for ET (see GES and EMET chapters) as well as to increase the number of embryos transferred to the uterus.

For women whose advancing age and/or ovarian resistance makes having a baby with their own eggs unappealing or unlikely, ovum donation (using donated eggs from a young donor, usually compatible and anonymous) is a highly successful option.

Approach to Ovarian Stimulation

As explained in chapter 5, the induction of ovulation with LH or hCG should be conducted against the backdrop of optimal follicle and egg development, and must occur at precisely the right time in order for the egg to achieve optimal maturation. Otherwise, the egg will be *dysmature* and unlikely to develop into a viable embryo capable of initiating a healthy implantation and pregnancy.

A potentially avoidable cause of poor egg development sometimes results through the injudicious use of stimulation protocols that fail to curtail the adverse influence of excessive LH and its effect on the overproduction of stromal male hormones (e.g., testosterone). This is especially the case in women who have raised basal FSH levels, women over 40, and women who have polycystic ovarian syndrome. It is thought that in such circumstances the incidence of structural and numerical chromosomal abnormalities occurring during meiosis could escalate. In this way the normal age-related incidence of egg aneuploidy may be further increased. Examples of a few stimulation protocols that we believe should preferably be avoided in such cases include the following: (1) GnRHa and gonadotropin stimulation initiated concurrently (i.e., microflare GnRHa protocols), (2) the use of clomiphene citrate, (3) a preponderance of LH-dominant gonadotropins (e.g., Repronex), and (4) late-follicular-phase GnRH-antagonist-gonadotropin protocols.

It is often claimed that women who develop ovarian hyperstimulation syndrome (OHSS) inherently have poor egg quality. This may not be the case. The fact is that such women, many of whom have PCOS (see chapter 5), have an inherent tendency to overproduce ovarian testosterone, placing them at increased risk of having poor-quality eggs. The tendency to prescribe high doses of LH-containing gonadotropins in such cases and to administer hCG prematurely in the hope of arresting further follicle growth and development so as to reduce the risk of OHSS often leads to poor egg development. The remedy is to allow the required time for optimal egg development to take place before giving hCG. The method whereby this is achieved is through prolonged coasting (see chapter 5).

IVF May Be the Only Way to Identify Inhibiting Factors in Eggs

Unexplained infertility is caused in many cases by some physical-chemical, biochemical, or immunological factors within the eggs that prevent the sperm from undergoing the acrosome reaction (being attracted to and then penetrating the zona pellucida). One way to determine whether such inhibiting factors might exist is by observing the interaction of eggs and sperm in the petri dish during IVF.

Expertise of the Embryology Team

It is sad yet true that when confronted with poor-quality eggs there is a tendency to lay the blame on the most convenient scapegoat, namely the embryologist(s). But in fact, poor embryology (deficient expertise, methodology, and technique) is rarely the cause of poor embryo quality and/or failed IVF. And most embryologists are much more disciplined and experienced in proven methodologies than are physicians.

QUALITY OF THE MAN'S SPERM: THE SECOND ULTIMATUM

Sperm DNA Integrity Assay (SDIA)

The important finding that DNA abnormalities in sperm, which can significantly reduce implantation and pregnancy rates, can be found in men with both normal and abnormal sperm counts, motility, and morphology led to the development of the sperm DNA integrity assay (SDIA) and the sperm chromatin structure assay (SCSA), both of which measure the same endpoints. The SDIA complements the standard semen analysis in evaluating sperm competency in preparation for IVF. (The SCSA will not be discussed here.)

Because DNA damage may be present in sperm from both fertile and infertile men, the SDIA may reveal a hidden abnormality of sperm DNA in men whose infertility previously had been classified as "unexplained." Infertile men with abnormal sperm characteristics exhibit increased levels of DNA damage in their sperm. Sperm from infertile men with normal-appearing sperm may have DNA damage to a degree comparable to that of infertile men with abnormal-appearing sperm. However, the data suggest that an abnormal SDIA is more likely to occur in cases of abnormal semen parameters.

Originally, most of the data available on the effects of abnormal SDIA results on fertility came from work performed using the SCSA in non-ART pregnancies. More recent data derived from IVF experience at SIRM suggests that the viable IVF pregnancy rate (thus, presumably, also the birthrate) is about two to three times lower in women whose partners have abnormal SDIAs. Results become progressively worse the older the woman gets.

We believe it is probably advantageous that an SDIA be performed prior to undertaking IVF/ICSI in cases where the sperm provider has not previously initiated a pregnancy that progressed beyond 12 weeks and/or where the man has an abnormal semen analysis.

In our experience, when the man has a concentration of healthy motile sperm of less than 10 million per ml, fertilization ability following conventional IVF (non-ICSI) begins to decline because the sperm's potential for fertilizing seems to be linked to the concentration of motile sperm. The normal concentration of motile sperm in any healthy male is about 50 percent or greater. Thus, if a man has a sperm count of 100 million per milliliter, he could expect to have 50 million motile sperm. New laboratory techniques for improving the motility of sperm, along with ICSI, offer renewed hope for men with even the severest forms of sperm dysfunction; in addition, new processing techniques in the laboratory facilitate the removal of some sperm antibodies that also may impact fertilization.

Sperm Antibodies

Strange as it may sound, a man can have antibodies to his own sperm. This is quite common after vasectomy, especially if there has been more than a eight-year interval since the procedure was done. The man might have a perfectly normal sperm count, motility, and morphology but the sperm may be coated with antibodies and may even clump or stick together, perhaps even precluding egg fertilization. Special laboratory techniques can partially overcome these problems.

QUALITY OF THE EMBRYO: THE THIRD ULTIMATUM

At this time, standard microscopic techniques for predicting the health and viability of embryos are far from optimal. Such limitations, coupled with pressure to maximize the chance of pregnancy, have typically resulted in a tendency to transfer too many embryos at a time. While such practice has led to improved IVF birthrates, the transfer of multiple embryos at one time has resulted in an unacceptably excessive rate of high-order multiple births (triplets or greater). This in turn has resulted in an alarming escalation in the incidence of prematurity-related neonatal complications that are all too often both life-threatening and life-enduring.

Of the approximately 3.5 million babies born annually in the U.S., about one in 500 is afflicted with a sex-linked disorder that occurs when a genetically defective Y (male) chromosome is transmitted to the offspring. Another one in 300 newborns has an autosomal genetic disorder, an abnormality of one or more genes involving the 44 remaining autosomes (non-sex chromosomes). This means that approximately one in 20,000 babies born annually in the U.S. will have one or another genetic or chromosomal disorder. In addition, about one in 50 babies is born with an identifiable major genetic abnormality. In other words, more than 70,000 babies are afflicted by severe genetic disease annually in this country. Many couples who parent a child with a severe birth defect will subsequently elect not to have another child and may adopt. These facts and figures offer a glimpse at the magnitude of the challenge confronting the medical profession, government, and society in general.

The Human Genome Project, a 15-year effort to draw the first detailed map in human DNA, will inevitably lead to the widespread implementation of human-gene therapy for the treatment and prevention of disease. We are on the verge of nothing less than a biomedical revolution the likes of which has not been encountered before. The human genome project will lead to profound changes in the ability to manipulate genes. It will change the way we are born, how we exist, how we view ourselves in relation to our destiny, and how we die.

Before us lies a difficult transition. Most people have begun to wonder about the cost; and while many are profoundly divided or even ambivalent about genetic research and its applications, most feel strongly that the introduction of human genetic engineering for the purpose of curing disease is well justified. If the use of genetic engineering to cure and prevent disease in an existing human being is justified, then surely the potential to eradicate certain lethal diseases through pre-implantation diagnosis is similarly vindicated.

Gender Selection

You may know someone who desperately wants to have a girl . . . or a boy. Perhaps a couple has several children of one gender already and would like to have another, but only if the odds of having a baby of the other gender could be greatly skewed in their favor. Or maybe the couple want a baby of one gender to avoid passing on one of the more than 500 sex-linked genetic diseases. Gender selection is discussed here because it can reduce the probability of X-linked diseases being passed on through the embryo.

Given that upon fertilization a sperm with a Y chromosome makes a boy and one bearing an X chromosome makes a girl, and any given sperm sample contains an even amount of X- and Y-bearing chromosomes, aspiring parents have no greater than a 50 percent chance of getting a baby of the desired sex. In ancient Greece, men believed that lying on their right side during intercourse increased the likelihood of a male child. A Chinese birth calendar buried over 700 years ago in a tomb outside Beijing is said to predict gender by when conception occurred. In 18th-century France, men would tie off their right testicle to "guarantee" having a boy. Sometimes, couples wanting a child of a particular gender use methods such as timing of intercourse. Until now, no method of gender selection has been shown to be scientifically valid.

A patented and proprietary preconception gender-selection process that uses a machine known as a flow cytometer to sort out sperm enriched in the desired gender is now available. The sperm are analyzed by the *fluorescence in situ hybridization* (FISH) process, in which the sperm are treated with a dye, which attaches temporarily to the DNA and fluoresces when exposed to laser light. Since the X chromosome is larger than the Y, the sperm with the X chromosomes will fluoresce more brightly than those with the Y. The flow cytometer is able to pick up these differences in brightness and separate the sperm as they move through the machine one at a time.

The Food and Drug Administration approved a clinical trial for this process, which is hoped to be completed by 2006. In order to qualify for the clinical trial, couples must currently be in one of two categories: (1) They must either have a history of one of the more than 500 X-linked diseases, where the woman is the known carrier (e.g., hemophilia and Duchenne muscular dystrophy; such couples may qualify for reduced-cost treatment) or (2) desire "family balancing" by sorting sperm for the less-represented sex of children in the family.

Sorted sperm can be used with various advanced reproductive techniques to achieve a pregnancy. The most common procedure is *intrauterine insemination* (IUI), in which the sperm is injected into the uterus by means of a catheter directed through the cervix, which enables sperm to reach and fertilize the egg more easily or to bypass hostile cervical mucus. (See discussion of IUI in chapter 10.) In preparation for IUI, the woman is monitored carefully to establish the time of ovulation, either by her local physician and/or at home with an ovulation-predictor kit. On the day that ovulation is expected to occur, the husband produces a sperm sample, the sperm are sorted for the desired gender, and the IUI with the sorted sperm occurs later that same day.

Using this method, there is about a 91 percent chance of having a female baby and about a 76 percent chance for a male. Based on the data so far, the likelihood of having a normal, healthy baby no matter which sex is not any different from that of the general population. As the technology continues to improve and becomes widely available, gender selection could become a more widely employed part of family planning.

The same technology can be used in conjunction with IVF and pre-implantation genetic diagnosis (PGD). An IVF cycle using sperm sorted by this technique should result in more embryos of the desired gender, and PGD testing can determine which embryos are female and which ones are male. If pregnancy results, there is almost a 100 percent chance the baby will be of the desired gender.

Preimplantation Genetic Diagnosis (PGD)

PGD is a technique used for the early diagnosis of chromosomal/genetic disorders in embryos or blastomeres (cells of the developing embryo). It involves conducting biopsies on the polar bodies of the embryo or upon a cell from the blastomere. PGD incorporates the latest techniques in assisted reproduction and molecular genetics to identify many chromosome/genetic disorders prior to the initiation of pregnancy, thereby providing real hope to many desperate couples who might transmit a potential genetic catastrophe to their offspring and negating the possible need for an abortion. Embryos shown to be free of the genetic disease under investigation thereupon can be selectively transferred to the uterus.

Polar body biopsy.   Polar body biopsy, which involves the removal of egg-derived chromosome populations known as polar bodies, can be performed relatively non-traumatically to the polar bodies within 36 hours of fertilization of the egg.

Blastomere biopsy.   Blastomere biopsy involves the removal of one or two blastomeres at the seven- to eight-cell stage of cleavage (day 3 after fertilization) and is performed for the purpose of diagnosing: (1) single or multiple gene disorders, (2) certain sex-linked genetic disorders, and (3) embryo aneuploidies involving the sex-chromosomes. It is also used to confirm the diagnosis of aneuploidy in cases where a polar biopsy produces a questionable result. Blastomere biopsy has two distinct advantages over polar body biopsy: (1) It allows investigative access to the genes located on the chromosomes, and (2) the application of FISH allows for the diagnosis of both egg and sperm-induced embryo aneuploidies. Additional reasons why blastomere biopsy is usually preferred over polar body biopsy are because a polar body is less likely to have optimal material for FISH, both polar bodies should be (but are not always) available for examination, and polar body biopsies look exclusively at the egg chromosomes and do not examine the contribution made by the sperm. Since about 10 percent of embryo aneuploidies can be traced to the sperm chromosomes, this renders the diagnosis of embryo aneuploidy less reliable. And for basically the same reason, polar body biopsies cannot determine embryo gender and thus will not allow for the pre-implantation diagnosis of sex-linked (Y-chromosome) disorders.

Unfortunately, PGD, as currently performed, commercially using FISH, can only evaluate nine out of a possible 23 chromosome pairs for aneuploidy. The aneuploidies responsible for poor embryo quality and reduced implantation potential are not necessarily the ones that involve the nine chromosome pairs that are presently tested through PGD using FISH. Thus, even if PGD were to reveal that the nine chromosome pairs evaluated were normal, it would not rule out embryo aneuploidy involving the remaining 14 chromosome pairs.

Furthermore, blastomere biopsy is a potentially traumatic process to the embryo and, as such, might reduce implantation potential of the normal embryo as tested. For these reasons, we believe that PGD for the purpose of excluding aneuploidy as a cause of "poor embryo quality" in an attempt to choose the "best embryos" for ET has limited (if any) value at present.

The prediction of genetic disorders using blastomere biopsy and *polymerase chain reaction* (PCR) technology, which involves identification and amplification of one or more gene loci on the chromosome, is expensive, requires the prior anticipation of an increased risk of the disorder occurring in the offspring, is very limited by the lack of availability of genetic markers for all but a handful of genetic diseases, and has little potential for widespread application or benefit.

Computerized genetic hybridization (CGH). CGH is a new technique involving the simultaneous evaluation of all chromosomes that could eventually find clinical application as a method of PGD. This could enable more accurate and complete diagnosis of existing embryo aneuploidies (structural as well as numerical), resulting in improved potential for confidently selecting fewer normal embryos for transfer. It is possible that CGH will ultimately replace FISH in the diagnosis of aneuploidy.

While there is good reason for optimism, it should be recognized that PGD is by no means 100 percent accurate. At the time of this writing, only 9 of the 23 chromosomal pairs were routinely evaluated by FISH. Thus, when a viable pregnancy occurs, a thorough prenatal genetic testing screen involving level-3 ultrasound examination, biochemical testing, and chorionic villus sampling (CVS)/mid-trimester amniocentesis should always be undertaken to exclude the risk of misdiagnosis through PGD.

UTERINE RECEPTIVITY: THE FOURTH ULTIMATUM

Contour of the Uterine Cavity

It has long been suspected that anatomical defects of the uterus might result in infertility. While fibroids confined to the uterine wall are unlikely to cause infertility, an association between their presence and infertility has been observed in cases where they distort the uterine cavity or protrude as submucous polyps through the endometrial lining. It would appear that even small submucous fibroids (ones that protrude into the uterine cavity) have the potential to prejudice implantation.

It is likely that any surface lesion in the uterine cavity, whether an endometrial, placental, or fibroid polyp (no matter how small) or intrauterine adhesion, has the potential to interfere with implantation by producing a local inflammatory response not too dissimilar in nature from that which is caused by a foreign body such as an intrauterine contraceptive device. Unfortunately, a hysterosalpingogram (HSG) will miss the diagnosis in approximately 30 percent of cases. The only reliable methods for diagnosing even the smallest of such lesions are fluid ultrasonography (FUS) or hysteroscopy.

If performed by an expert, FUS is highly effective in recognizing even the smallest lesion and can replace hysteroscopy under such circumstances. FUS is also less expensive and less traumatic. Its only disadvantage lies in the fact that if a lesion is detected, the subsequent performance of hysteroscopy may be required to treat the problem. Diagnostic hysteroscopy involves the insertion of a thin, lighted, telescope-like hysteroscope into the uterus, which is first distended with a sterile solution or with carbon dioxide gas. As is the case with FUS, diagnostic hysteroscopy facilitates examination of the inside of the uterus under direct vision for defects that might interfere with implantation. We have observed that approximately one in 10 candidates for IVF has lesions that require attention prior to undergoing IVF in order to optimize the chances of a successful outcome. We strongly recommend that all patients undergo therapeutic surgery (usually by hysteroscopy) to correct the pathology.

Thickness of the Endometrium

The importance of the quality of the endometrium and its potential to promote implantation cannot be overstated. When the zona pellucida breaks open and out burst the cells, which try to sink their way into the lining of the uterine wall, whether this embryo is unable to implant, implants but has stunted growth, or grows into a healthy baby, depends on the quality of the endometrium.

In 1989, we were first to show that in both normal and stimulated cycles, preovulatory endometrial thickness/ultrasound appearance is predictive of embryo implantation potential following IVF. With conventional IVF there needs to be a 9 mm sagital thickness (Grade 2) and a triple line appearance (Grade A) of the endometrium. Accordingly, a Grade 2A lining is optimal in such cases. Anything less is associated with a significant reduction in live birthrates per ET. A possible exception may apply in cases of third-party embryo recipients (e.g., ovum donation, IVF-surrogacy, and frozen embryo transfers, in which the recipient receives supplementary estrogen/progesterone and not gonadotropins to prepare the uterine lining). Here, a lining 8 mm thick may be adequate.

A poor endometrial lining most commonly occurs in women with a history of unexplained recurrent IVF failures or early recurrent miscarriages and is usually attributable to (1) inflammation of the endometrium (i.e., endometritis occurring following a septic delivery, abortion, or miscarriage), (2) adenomyosis (gross invasion of the uterine muscle by endometrial glandular tissue), (3) multiple fibroid tumors of the endometrium, (4) prenatal exposure to the synthetic hormone diethylstilbestrol (DES), and (5) administration of clomiphene citrate for at least three consecutive months without a resting cycle (this effect is self-reversible within four to six weeks of discontinuing clomiphene).

Attempts to augment poor endometrial linings by bolstering circulating blood estrogen levels through increased doses of fertility drugs, aspirin, and by supplementary estrogen therapy have yielded disappointing results. We reported on the ability of vaginally administered Viagra and the addition of oral beta adrenergic agents (e.g., Terbutaline or Ritodrine) to significantly enhance uterine blood flow and estrogen delivery to the endometrium, thereby improving its development and facilitating healthy pregnancies.

If an assessment reveals the endometrium to be poor, the woman should probably opt out of that particular cycle of IVF. She then has three choices: Her eggs can be removed, fertilized, and frozen for the purpose of transferring them to the uterus in a subsequent cycle when she has been treated with Viagra hormonal replacement; she can return for a fresh cycle while Viagra vaginal therapy is used; or her embryos can be transferred into the uterus of a surrogate.

The Immunology Factor

Antibodies are proteins that are made by the immune system as a primary defense against infection and injury by foreign proteins. (The immune system is able to distinguish between proteins that are "self" and those which are foreign, or "nonself.")

Normally, the immune systems of most women will not react against sperm; but in some cases, for unknown reasons, antibodies are produced that deactivate sperm. In addition, because the immunologic imprint of the implanting conceptus (the implanted embryo and/or early fetus) is comprised of immunological factors contributed by both the woman and her partner, and the man's imprint is immunologically foreign to the woman, it is surprising that women don't summarily reject all pregnancies. This is sometimes referred to as "the immunologic riddle of pregnancy."

Alloimmunity. The woman's ability to successfully host a pregnancy depends largely upon a complex interplay of sophisticated immunologic adjustments designed to convert her uterus to a privileged site that would protect the developing conceptus from rejection. The relevant imprints of the man's immunologic makeup (reflected in his sperm) differ substantially from those of the woman, and her immune system recognizes the immunologic difference as soon as the embryo attempts to implant itself into the endometrium. In response, she produces *antipaternal lymphocyte antibodies* (APLA) against specific sperm-related antigens to protect the conceptus from those components of her immune system that would otherwise attack. This quarantines the embryo, protecting it from rejection. But sometimes these mechanisms can go wrong; and depending upon when this happens, the woman might experience repeated pregnancy loss.

The production of such APLA is referred to as an *alloimmune response.* In cases where the man and woman share the same antigens, the required alloimmune response may be inadequate or completely fail to take place. Thus, sufficient APLA might not develop, thereby exposing the conceptus to rejection. Depending on the severity and timing of the failed alloimmune process, implantation could fail so early that the woman would not even know she was pregnant. However, this is rarely a cause of early implantation failure. Rather, an inadequate alloimmune response is much more likely to produce recurrent miscarriage, a later pregnancy loss, or retarded growth of the baby (a complication of pregnancy relating to poor development of the placenta).

Autoimmunity.   In some circumstances, antibodies develop to the body's own cell components. This is known as autoimmunity. In some autoimmune diseases these antibodies cause the body to reject its own tissues. Examples include rheumatoid arthritis, lupus erythematosis, and hypothyroidism. It is perhaps not surprising that these conditions are commonly associated with repeated pregnancy failure and loss.

Antiphospholipid antibodies (APA).   A large body of literature has confirmed that patients who experience repeated IVF failures often have increased levels of circulating APAs. Compelling evidence has also demonstrated that 30–50 percent of women with pelvic endometriosis and unexplained infertility harbor APAs in their blood. Despite this information, the role of APAs in reproductive outcome is still controversial. In 1995, we proposed that in cases of *non-male-factor infertility,* women who test positive for APAs be treated with minidose heparin to improve IVF implantation and thus birthrates. This approach was based upon research that suggested that heparin repels APAs from the surface of trophoblast cells, thus enhancing their development. We subsequently demonstrated that heparin therapy improved IVF outcome only in cases where the women tested positive for IgG and/or

IgM APAs other than two types of phospholipids, namely, anti-phosphatidylethanolamine (aPE) and anti-phosphatidylserine (aPS). Women who had IgG/IgM-related anti-PE or anti-PS antibodies only experienced a significant improvement in IVF implantation and birthrates when intravenous immunoglobulin (IVIG) therapy (discussed later) was given beginning seven to 10 days prior to embryo transfer.

Notwithstanding the above, the following recent observations suggest that APAs, rather than being causally linked to implantation failure, might serve to identify a population at inordinate risk of implantation failure and that cytotoxic/activated (NKa) cells and T-cells (see next subsection), through the unregulated release of toxins, are in fact the real culprits. In addition, it has been determined that the presence of APAs in male-factor cases appears to bear no relationship to IVF outcome; only APA-positive women who also test positive for NKa and/or T-cell activation appear to benefit from selective immunotherapy with IVIG. We observed that more than 75 percent of women testing positive for APA who have in addition increased NKa also harbor anti-PE and/or anti-PS antibodies.

Administration of low-dose heparin to APA-positive women who test negative for NKa or T-cell activation essentially doubles the pregnancy rate. Should women who have APA conceive, the treatment continues through the first 10 weeks of the pregnancy.

Natural killer (NK) and T-cell cytotoxicity. After ovulation and during early pregnancy, NK cells comprise more than 80 percent of the white blood cell population seen in the uterine lining. NK cells produce a variety of local hormones known as TH-1 cytokines ("embryotoxic factor"). Uncontrolled, excessive release of TH-1 cytokines is highly toxic to the trophoblast and endometrial cells, leading to their programmed death and, subsequently, to failed implantation. Activated NK cells (NKa) can spill over from the uterine lining into the peripheral blood, where their toxicity can be measured. In the following situations these NK cells (and also T-cells) can become abnormally activated (NKa), and thereby overproduce TH-1 cytokines: (1) in female patients who have both pelvic disease (especially endometriosis, regardless of severity) and abnormal APA testing, and (2) in about half of cases where the woman forms antibodies against her own thyroid gland (i.e., antithyroid antibodies). IVIG therapy, initiated one to two weeks prior to embryo transfer, can subdue NKa cells, thereby reducing the risk of implantation failure.

Antithyroid antibodies (ATA). The production of antithyroid autoantibodies to women's thyroid glands may occur regardless of whether or not there are clinical signs or symptoms of reduced thyroid hormone activity (hypothyroidism), although one of the most significant hints that a non-symptomatic woman might have ATA is a family history of hypothyroidism. Antithyroid antibodies probably do not directly attack the embryo or fetus. Instead, they likely act as "markers" pointing to an underlying tendency toward rejection of the embryo or fetus through an allergic type (hypersensitivity) response. Here, as soon as the embryo starts to burrow into the uterine wall, toxins are produced (locally) that impair implantation. In some cases, the pregnancy is lost before a blood test can detect it, while in other cases a miscarriage occurs. (Some pregnancies escape the "toxic gauntlet" and proceed.) The presence of antithyroid antibodies is associated with a variety of manifestations of poor reproductive performance, ranging from infertility through miscarriages to later pregnancy complications, such as intrauterine growth retardation, fetal death, and prematurity. About 50 percent of women who harbor ATAs, regardless of whether or not they have clinical hypothryoidism, demonstrate the presence of activated T-cells and/or NKa, and require IVIG therapy.

Activated T-cells. T-cells are involved in the cellular-immune or delayed hypersensitivity response. Activated T-cells release toxins that accelerate destruction of the early embryo's root system. Studies have shown that women who experience recurrent pregnancy loss often have a high concentration of activated T-cells, NKa cells, and raised endometrial and blood levels of TH-1 cytokines. The administration of IVIG with corticosteroids such as Dexamethazone suppress the activity of T-cells.

Immunologic implantation failure: treatment options.

Heparin. There is compelling evidence that subcutaneous minidose heparin administration to women undergoing IVF for female causes of infertility who test positive for APAs, but negative for NKa, significantly improves IVF birthrates. Heparin is thought to act by repelling APAs from the surface of the trophoblast. Provided that the woman's platelet count remains normal and heparin is withheld on the day of egg retrieval, its administration is virtually risk-free. In the past we prescribed aspirin in combination with minidose heparin in cases of APA positivity, but evidence now indicates that the administration of aspirin in combination with heparin offers no tangible benefit over treatment with heparin alone for the management of such IVF patients. With the possible exception of women with primary APA-related autoimmune diseases (e.g., lupus erythematosis, rheumatoid arthritis, dermatomyositis, scleroderma, etc.) and in cases associated with recurrent pregnancy loss, we no longer prescribe aspirin to women undergoing treatment for reproductive failure.

Intravenous immunoglobulin (IVIG). IVIG is a sterile protein preparation derived from human blood that is as free as possible from bacterial and viral contamination. There are several ways in which IVIG may offset or counter the anti-implantation effects associated with reproductive immunologic deficiencies: (1) It is a potent suppressor of toxic NKa cells; (2) it contains anti-idiotype antibodies that combat the effects of harmful antibodies, thereby protecting the embryo/fetus from rejection; and (3) it deactivates activated T-cells that may be involved in poor reproductive performance.

Unfortunately, IVIG has had some undeserved bad press. Since it is a blood derivative, the thought of administering it in an era where HIV is rampant is frightening to many. But consider the following: The IVIG products available in the United States and the United Kingdom have not, according to the manufacturers, resulted in a single HIV viral transmission in millions of administrations. Moreover, IVIG is derived from the very same blood pool used for transfusion purposes; millions of units of blood have been administered in the United States over the last 10 years without any reports of HIV transmission, and the product is thoroughly tested in the United States. Local manufacturers claim that US-produced IVIG is untainted by viral contamination. IVIG therapy for increased NKa/T-cell activation should be initiated at least seven to 10 days prior to embryo transfer.

The infusion is usually repeated once pregnancy has been diagnosed through the performance of serial Beta hCG blood tests. Thereafter, with a few notable exceptions, IVIG therapy is canceled for the remainder of the pregnancy.

Corticosteroid therapy (Prednisone, Prenisilone, and Dexamethazone). Corticosteroid therapy is a mainstay of most IVF programs. Some programs use daily oral methyl prednisilone (Medrol), while we and others prescribe oral Dexamethazone commencing about 10 days prior to initiating ovarian stimulation with gonadotropins and continuing until the eighth week of pregnancy or until pregnancy is discounted, where upon the dosage is tapered off over a period of seven to 10 days and then discontinued. Corticosteroids are believed to act by inhibiting the cellular immune response and thereby improving embryo implantation potential.

The selective use of immunotherapy has, on numerous occasions, enabled us to achieve successful pregnancies in patients who had previously suffered four or more IVF failures. Many such patients had been advised not to try again with their own eggs. We are able to report numerous IVF births occurring after more than 10 prior IVF failures. It is indisputable that such results would not have been achieved without access to selective immunotherapy. We have been able to demonstrate that NKa and T-cell-activated women who do not receive IVIG therapy have a 15-fold reduction in the chance of successful IVF.

Given the potential roles of immunologic problems in pregnancy and IVF, it is important to properly evaluate all women who have the following risk factors for such problems before they undergo IVF: (1) unexplained or recurrent IVF failures, (2) endometriosis (about 33 percent of cases are associated with increased NKa, requiring IVIG therapy), (3) unexplained infertility, (4) infertility following recurrent miscarriage, and (5) personal or family history of autoimmune disorders such as rheumatoid arthritis, lupus erythematosis, and hypothyroidism (or Hashimoto's disease, which occurs more often in women).

Infective organisms. Finally, the presence of organisms that negatively impact implantation should be ruled out prior to IVF. Except for ureaplasma, the presence of these organisms is indicated by their symptoms. Ureaplasma rarely presents symptoms, although occasionally it may produce a poor postcoital test (see chapter 10).

EMBRYO TRANSFER: THE FIFTH ULTIMATUM

It cannot be overstated that embryo transfer is the single most determinant factor in IVF outcome. The procedure requires gentle placement of the embryo(s) within 1 cm of the roof of the uterine cavity under direct ultrasound visualization.

The selection of embryos most likely to implant and the timing of embryo transfer, both critical to the transfer process, have been greatly enhanced by use of the following three elements in the embryo transfer protocol: Graduated Embryo Scoring (GES), blastocyst transfer, and the Embryo Marker Expression Test (EMET). Both GES and EMET were developed by SIRM and are used at all the SIRM clinics.

Graduated Embryo Scoring (GES)

Graduated Embryo Scoring (GES) is a unique microscopic method for assessing embryo quality. With GES, each embryo is separately examined through a series of microscopic assessments throughout a period of 72 hours following egg insemination. The maximum allotted GES score is 100. A four-year evaluation of embryos derived from the eggs of thousands of women under 40 has revealed that embryos with a GES score of 70–100 each have better than a 35 percent likelihood of implanting successfully as compared to less than 20 percent when the GES score is below 70. Embryo implantation potential decreases rapidly, progressively, and proportionately to well below 10 percent per embryo by the time the egg provider reaches 43 years of age.

It was largely the need to grow embryos separately in order to implement GES throughout all SIRM centers that led to our discovering that the presence of sHLA-G in the media surrounding each embryo could predict which embryos were most likely to produce a pregnancy (see "The Embryo Marker Expression Test (EMET)" later in this section). At the time of this writing, almost all other IVF programs were growing embryos in batches (more than one embryo in the same petri dish).

Blastocyst Transfer

The presumption has always been that it is better to transfer healthy embryos into the uterus sooner rather than later once the best ones for transfer have been identified. It is against this background that attention has been focused on the transfer of more-developed embryos (blastocyst stage). Since the late 1990s, this process, known as *blastocyst transfer* (BT), has become increasingly prevalent among ART programs. The transfer of good-quality blastocysts is associated with a high rate of pregnancy, but it carries with it the risk of high-order multiple pregnancies unless fewer blastocysts are transferred because they are considered likely to implant.

Prior to the first cell-division, the freshly fertilized pre-embryo displays two pronuclei, one derived from each parent, and which contain the genetic material. From 24 to 30 hours after fertilization (day one), the embryo should have divided into two cells, by day two it should have four cells, and by day three, there should be seven to eight cells. Until day three, all the cells are identical. Embryonic development is controlled by maternal genes in the egg until around the eight-cell stage, when the potential for further development comes under the control of the embryo itself. By day five the cells have started to differentiate into specific types, each with a specialized function. The outer cells will eventually form the placenta and fetal membranes. Secretions from inner cells collect in a central cavity, called the blastocele, and become the amniotic fluid. Specialized cells on the inner surface of the morula form the *inner cell mass* (ICM) that eventually develops into the fetus. This complex creation is now called a blastocyst. As the cavity fills with fluid, the blastocyst expands and eventually "hatches" from the zona pellucida. The hatched blastocyst then implants into the endometrium six to seven days after ovulation.

Human embryos have specific metabolic requirements in order to survive and develop optimally. Fertilization normally occurs in the fallopian tube, which is a metabolically distinct environment, having less oxygen and less glucose than the uterus. Early IVF culture media, which inadequately replicated this tubal environment, could only support limited embryonic development; most embryos survived only to the cleavage stage. Improved culture media, which resulted in reliable embryo survival to day three, has been the standard in many programs since approximately 1994. In 1997, researchers in Australia, Scandinavia, and the United States concurrently developed a new generation of culture media that can reliably support embryo growth until day five to six. This improved culture media, based on the premise that the metabolic needs of the early embryo change as it moves from the fallopian tube to the uterus, more closely mimics the body's environment. Now approximately 50 percent of good-quality day three embryos (seven to eight cells) can be grown to the blastocyst stage, which has made blastocyst transfer widely available throughout the world.

The major benefit from extending embryo culture to day five is a natural selection of the best-quality embryos. This means high pregnancy rates can be achieved from the transfer of fewer embryos than usual, thus reducing the risk of high-order multiple pregnancies. It is possible in patients with multiple good-appearing embryos on day three that poor-quality embryos could be selected for transfer to the uterus by pure chance. For this reason, more embryos are usually transferred when ET is performed on day three, again increasing the risk of a high-order multiple gestation.

By culturing the embryos for an additional 48 hours, many of the suboptimal ones do not survive, leaving only the best embryos to select from on day five. Unfortunately, some women will not have any embryos survive to day five despite that they appeared healthy on day three. While it is highly likely that those embryos that do not survive to the blastocyst stage in culture are not strong enough to survive in the natural uterine environment either, this still remains to be proven conclusively. Blastocyst transfer is probably of questionable benefit in women with suboptimal embryos on day three.

It has long been thought that an embryo that develops rapidly is more likely to implant successfully, although overly rapid growth (more than 10 cells on day three) is associated with decreased pregnancy rates. It is also well established that poor-quality embryos tend to develop slower and are much more likely to arrest before reaching the blastocyst stage than normal-quality ones. In this sense, extended embryo culture to day five can be used as a type of "biologic assay" to help select the best-quality embryos for transfer.

At SIRM as well as in a growing number of other IVF centers, embryos are now cultured individually (rather than in batches) so as to permit monitoring the developmental progression of each embryo separately. This cannot be done when embryos are batched and cultured together. By evaluating the achievement of certain critical developmental milestones, it has been possible for us to predict on day three with a good degree of certainty which embryos are likely to survive until day five, which has allowed the high pregnancy rates associated with BT transfer from day three-ET. In fact, early embryo scoring has made extended embryo culture unnecessary for the majority of couples in our program.

It is important not to lose sight of the fact that the optimal goal of fertility treatment is to recreate the natural situation of a singleton gestation. As our knowledge of embryo development increases, so will our ability to select embryos with a good prognosis for causing a pregnancy. In the foreseeable future, it is very likely that we will be able to achieve high pregnancy rates from the transfer of a single embryo. Until that time, extended embryo culture and/or early embryo grading are the best tools available to identify those embryos most likely to implant.

The material in this section was provided by Jeffrey D. Fisch, M.D., of the Sher Institute for Reproductive Medicine—Las Vegas, Nevada.

The Embryo Marker Expression Test (EMET)

By measuring the concentration of a genetic marker known as *sHLA-G* (soluble human leukocyte antigen-G), which is released into the media in which early embryos are growing after fertilization, it is now possible to identify those embryos most likely to produce a pregnancy. The Embryo Marker Expression Test (EMET) is performed 46 hours after the egg retrieval to identify EMET-positive, or "competent" embryos. It has been determined, based upon the performance of EMET in more than 500 women undergoing IVF at SIRM, that the transfer of even a *single* EMET-positive embryo in women under 39 (provided that they had normal uterine linings and, when needed, were treated for immunologic implantation problems) results in better than a 60 percent chance of a viable pregnancy. Comparable results in women 39–43 years was above 40 percent. The transfer of more than one EMET-positive embryo at a time resulted in a great increase in the multiple pregnancy rate without significantly improving the overall pregnancy rate.

We conclude that measurement of sHLA-G in the media surrounding two-day-old embryos in order to select competent embryos allows for a reduction in the number of embryos transferred on day three, thereby minimizing the risk of high-order multiple pregnancies (triplets or greater) while optimizing IVF success.

This discovery is changing the way IVF is performed by bringing IVF practitioners much closer to the long-awaited objective of "one embryo, one healthy baby."

Perhaps equally important is that now, by measuring sHLA-G (and perhaps similar molecular markers, as yet unidentified) produced by early embryos, we can establish a rational basis by which we can customize protocols used for ovarian stimulation to better meet the needs of separate categories of patients and so measurably improve egg/embryo quality and IVF success rates. Just as one size of any garment will not fit everyone, so no single regimen of ovarian stimulation is adequate for all patients. The use of biochemical and genetic markers of "embryo competency" such as sHLA-G could also provide researchers as well as the pharmaceutical industry with a method that would help in the development of new and more efficacious fertility drugs that produce fewer side effects with reduced risk to patients.

It is hoped that the proof that such advances can improve IVF outcome—and reduce risk as well as virtually eliminate high-order multiple pregnancies—will prompt health insurance companies to revisit the issue of universal infertility coverage. Until then, the size of the pocket book still determines the ability to go from infertility to family.

The above sections on GES, blastocyst transfer, and EMET provide an overview of the means by which the embryos most likely to implant are selected and nurtured at SIRM. How these elements are mixed and matched varies according to individual circumstances. Although it is not possible to generalize how they would be used, the following situations are examples of what might occur before embryo transfer. In the case of embryos scoring 70 or higher, we might advise culturing them to blastocyst stage; but at other times we would add one or two poorer-scoring embryos to a 70+ one and transfer on day 3 post–egg retrieval. If there are only a few embryos and all score below 70, we might transfer several at once in the hope that one might implant; but if there are many embryos scoring below 70, we might culture them two to three days longer to test if they will go to blastocyst stage. Presently EMET is available to all women doing IVF at SIRM. EMET, once requested by a woman/couple, is performed on all divided embryos on day 2 (i.e., one day prior to establishing the final GES score and transferring embryos). Thus, the EMET result influences which embryos are chosen, usually overriding the GES parameters. Each case must be evaluated individually. This is an example how a merger of the "art" and the "science" of IVF can profoundly benefit the woman and her partner.

The Role of Preimplantation Genetic Diagnosis (PGD) in Selecting the Best Embryos for Transfer

Currently, probes used in fluorescence in-situ hybridization (FISH) only examine eight or nine of the 23 human chromosome pairs in the embryo. Thus, most chromosome pairs cannot be examined for numerical chromosome abnormalities (aneuploidy). The eight or nine commercially available probes were actually developed to test for the most common aneuploidies that cause chromosomal miscarriages and birth defects. Since FISH as performed commercially at the time of this writing will not evaluate for many "lethal aneuploidies," it is of very limited value in selecting chromosomally normal embryos for transfer. Furthermore, because PGD does not measure the sHLA-G produced by the embryos in the culture media, it is of no use in identifying competent embryos. (See discussion of PGD earlier in this chapter in "Quality of the Embryo: The Third Ultimatum.")

Individuals and/or couples who do not meet all the above-mentioned ultimatums should not necessarily despair. Depending on the couple's particular set of circumstances, the physician, assisted by a first-rate IVF laboratory, can compensate for the lack of or deficiency in some of the criteria by employing today's high-tech procedures. For example, although both the number and quality of eggs tend to decrease with age, a woman over 40 with a large, healthy uterus and the proper hormonal environment may become pregnant even if the laboratory is able to fertilize only one or two eggs. (See Chapter 12 for suggested ways in which couples can estimate their IVF outcome although they do not fulfill all the ultimatums to the letter.)

9

OTHER CONDITIONS THAT NEGATIVELY IMPACT FERTILITY

CONDITIONS THAT NEGATIVELY IMPACT A MAN'S FERTILITY

Inadequate Secretion by the Pituitary Gland

In a relatively small number of cases of male infertility, the failure to produce an adequate quality of sperm relates to reduced secretion by the pituitary gland of those hormones necessary to stimulate sperm production. The pituitary gland in the man produces two important hormones with regard to testicular function: follicle-stimulating hormone (FSH) and luteinizing hormone (LH). LH's predominant function is to act on the Leydig cells in the testicles, which produce the male hormone testosterone. A sustained reduction in FSH production, therefore, is capable of resulting in male infertility. Usually, if there is a reduction in either LH or FSH, the other one will also be low. Men produce sperm in cycles of approximately 90 to 100 days, from initiation to the production of the most mature forms of sperm. Accordingly, any treatment administered to the man in order to improve sperm production can only be properly assessed after waiting about three months. In order to assess the potential of a male to respond to fertility drugs, it is therefore necessary to first measure both FSH and LH as well as the male hormones testosterone, androstenedione, dehydroepiandrosterone, and prolactin. Measurement of these hormones gives an indication as to whether the man is likely to respond to treatment with FSH or FSH/LH.

There are three approaches to treating male infertility that are potentially responsive to therapy:

Clomiphene citrate.   As mentioned earlier, clomiphene citrate is a hormone that stimulates the pituitary gland to produce large amounts of FSH and LH, which is essential to the production of sperm. The first step in this simple treatment is to perform a baseline semen analysis, FSH, LH, and male hormone measurements immediately prior to initiating therapy. Then 25 mg of clomiphene citrate is administered every other day for 100 days, and all of the tests are repeated serially throughout the treatment period. The administration of clomiphene citrate is essentially harmless to the man, who may experience some minor side effects such as spots in front of the eyes, dryness of the mouth, headaches, slight changes in mood, and, rarely, hot flashes. All of these side effects abate upon discontinuation of therapy.

Gonadotropin therapy.   In cases where clomiphene citrate therapy is not successful or in certain situations where it is not possible for clomiphene to stimulate the pituitary gland into action, FSH alone or in combination with LH can be administered in the hope of stimulating the testicles directly. This therapy might also include the administration of hCG in order to further stimulate the production of male hormones in cases where failed masculinization is associated with reduced sperm production. These drugs are usually administered three times per week, again for about 100 days, and the same hormonal and sperm assessments as stipulated for clomiphene therapy would apply. The treatment is, again, relatively harmless, and the minor side effects that might occur cease upon discontinuation of therapy.

Other medical therapies.   There is some evidence that the administration of certain vitamin preparations and antioxidants are of benefit in the treatment of male infertility associated with an abnormal SDIA and/or reduced sperm motility.

In some cases, systemic conditions affecting other areas of the body might indirectly impact upon the pituitary gland's ability to produce the hormones necessary to stimulate testicular function. In cases of thyroid deficiency, severe diabetes mellitus, and collagen diseases, selective therapy with thyroid hormone, insulin, or corticosteroids may be of benefit. Sometimes the pituitary gland produces too much prolactin, which in turn inhibits the ability of FSH and LH to act on the testicles. In such cases, it may be necessary to administer a drug called Parlodel (bromocriptine) to suppress prolactin production, thereby removing its restraining effect on the action of FSH upon the testicles. There are, of course, many other such examples in which treatment of unrelated conditions might improve overall male fertility. Such approaches as the use of temperature-lowering devices on the testicles and prevention of exposure to dangerous chemicals have been reported to be preventative and even curative, but in our opinion they are of dubious value.

If the previously infertile man is indeed fortunate enough to respond to one of the above treatment modalities for enhancement of sperm production, then it is possible for a number of masturbation specimens of sperm to be collected and frozen in liquid nitrogen so there will always be relatively good-quality sperm on hand, even if the fertility treatment is discontinued and the man again produces relatively poor sperm. It is, of course, not practical to permanently treat an individual on potent medications such as clomiphene, FSH, LH, or hCG.

CONDITIONS THAT NEGATIVELY IMPACT A WOMAN'S FERTILITY

Pelvic Inflammatory Disease (PID)

Pelvic inflammatory disease (PID) results from infection of pelvic structures, especially the fallopian tubes, via which the uterus, fallopian tubes, ovaries, bowel, and the smooth membrane that lines the surface of the pelvic cavity (the peritoneum) may also be infected. PID's damage to pelvic structures can inhibit the passage of eggs, sperm, and embryos in a timely manner to and from the uterine cavity, thus compromising fertility.

It has been estimated that about 1.2 million women develop PID annually in the United States. Less than one-third of these women present with acute pelvic inflammatory disease, and the remaining cases usually go undetected until the woman presents with symptoms of infertility. In fact, more than 60 percent of patients who undergo surgery or IVF are unaware of any history of acute PID. It is an unfortunate irony that although many of the sexually transmitted organisms are readily eradicated through appropriate antibiotic therapy, because their presence produces no overt symptoms women thus infected rarely seek treatment.

Grades of severity.   *Acute PID* usually prompts the woman to seek immediate medical attention because of fever, severe lower abdominal pain, a yellow- or blood-stained nonirritating vaginal discharge, and vomiting. More commonly, the onset of *sub-acute PID* is gradual, less severe, and often goes unnoticed until superimposed acute PID occurs or chronic incapacitating symptoms prompt the woman to seek medical attention. *Chronic PID,* a consequence of untreated or unsuccessfully managed acute and/or subacute PID, presents with symptoms of pelvic pain, heavy and painful menstrual periods, pain with intercourse, and infertility.

Causes.   PID results from (1) sexual transmission via the vagina and cervix of infecting organisms, (2) contamination from other inflamed structures in the abdominal cavity (e.g., appendix, gallbladder, kidneys, etc.), (3) a foreign body inside the uterus (e.g., an IUD), (4) contamination of retained products of conception following abortion or childbirth, and, rarely, (5) blood-borne bacterial transmission (e.g., pelvic tuberculosis, which is common in developing countries but rare in the United States).

Factors that facilitate development of PID include (1) exposure to infection immediately prior to menstruation because menstrual blood provides an excellent growth medium for bacteria, (2) relatively ill health and poor nutritional status, which is why PID is rampant in lower socioeconomic groups, and (3) high susceptibility to re-infection of women with a history of PID. While sexually transmitted PID is certainly capable of causing *endometritis* (infection of the uterine lining), the fallopian tubes rather than the uterus itself are usually the main focus of the inflammatory process in such cases because menstruation tends to remove infected tissue monthly, thereby preventing the inflammation from causing permanent damage to the endometrium.

In contrast, PID that occurs following childbirth or abortion primarily targets the uterine lining because the delayed onset of menstruation after both childbirth and abortion enables the inflammatory process to take hold in the products of conception that are sometimes retained in the uterus. This sometimes leads to the development of scar tissue in the uterine cavity and can cause opposing surfaces of the endometrium to fuse (Asherman's syndrome); produce scarring that obliterates the junction into the fallopian tubes and might also damage a small, adjacent segment of the tubes; and cause the fallopian tube(s) to separate from the uterine wall. Less commonly, post-childbirth and post-abortal endometritis can result in *salpingitis,* or infection of the entire fallopian tube(s), causing partial or complete blockage and/or spreading into the pelvic cavity.

PID may also result from the use of the intrauterine contraceptive device (IUD) for contraceptive purposes. This most commonly occurs in cases where the device is inserted into the uterus of women concurrently infected with gonorrhea or chlamydia. The IUD causes local irritation that compromises the defense mechanisms normally protecting against infection. At the same time, the IUD string, which protrudes through the cervix into the vagina, may act as a wick via which infecting organisms gain entrance to the uterus. IUD-related uterine infection causes the same damage as post-abortal and post-childbirth endometritis. IUD-related PID is a potentially life-endangering condition capable of causing formation of a pelvic abscess, peritonitis, systemic infection, and shock.

In cases where the ends of the fallopian tubes are blocked, pus may collect and distend the tube(s). The pus is usually absorbed over time and replaced by clear straw-colored fluid, resulting in occluded, fluid-filled, distended, and often functionless fallopian tube(s), referred to as a *hydrosalpinx.* This fluid, which contains dead cells and other noxious products, is believed to be toxic to embryos and can hinder implantation following IVF. Difficult as it may be to accept, women with hydrosalpinges should strongly consider having their tubes removed or ligated prior to undergoing IVF. This is because the presence of hydrosalpinges renders the tubes non-functional; and even if the tubes could be opened, the likelihood of pregnancy occurring would be remote.

Sexually transmitted PID almost invariably affects both fallopian tubes. Even in cases where hysterosalpingogram or laparoscopy (see explanation of tests in the following chapter) indicates that only one fallopian tube has been infected, the other tube is almost invariably involved. A procedure called *tuboscopy* (where a thin fiber-optic telescope is passed into the fallopian tube(s) to evaluate the inner structure) has confirmed that the tubes of women with a history of PID, who seemingly have normal pelvic anatomy, oftentimes have previously undetected internal scarring and/or adhesions.

Pelvic Tuberculosis

Pelvic tuberculosis is an uncommon cause of infertility in the United States although its incidence is on the rise as a result of the influx of immigrants from Asia, particularly India, and other underdeveloped countries where poor nutrition and general ill health contribute to its formation.

Pelvic tuberculosis is often a "silent disease" that may exist for 10 to 20 years without producing any symptoms. Infertility is often one of the reasons—and sometimes the only reason—to investigate for the presence of the condition; and because of its rarity as a cause of infertility in the United States, the diagnosis is often missed.

Pelvic tuberculosis usually presents with one or more of the following symptoms: (1) pelvic pain, pain with menstruation, pain with intercourse, chronic lower abdominal pain or discomfort, chronic back pain; (2) abdominal distention, usually due to the collection of free fluid in the abdominal-pelvic cavity; (3) local tuberculous lesions on the external genitalia, cervix, and/or vagina; (4) tuberculous salpingitis (tubal disease), which occurs in 75 percent of cases; (5) ovulation dysfunction, which often presents with absent, excessive, or noncyclical menstruation, largely attributable to ovarian involvement (40 percent of cases); and (6) uterine (endometrial) tuberculosis (30 percent).

Diagnosis. The diagnosis is made on the basis of evidence of concomitant, pulmonary tuberculosis; the detection of calcifications on pelvic X-rays; a typical tubal pattern on hysterosalpingogram (dye X-ray test); findings at laparoscopy or laparotomy and the subsequent pathologic examination of biopsy material obtained during these procedures; and blood tests such as a differential blood count and erythrocyte sedimentation rate.

Microscopic and bacteriologic examination is the primary method for diagnosing pelvic tuberculosis. Most commonly, a dilatation and curettage (D&C) of the uterus is performed a few days prior to menstruation. The surgeon uses a physiologic salt solution to cleanse the vagina and cervix while preparing for the D&C lest an antiseptic kill any tuberculous bacilli present in the specimen, thereby rendering a falsely negative culture result. Upon collection, part of the specimen of uterine curettings is cultured by the bacteriologic lab and some is used for guinea pig inoculation for detection of the acid-fast tuberculosis. Biopsy specimens of lesions on the external genitalia, vagina, cervix, and pelvic cavity can also be studied by culturing, by guinea pig inoculation, and by histopathologic examination. Even in the presence of established tuberculosis, histopathologic examination will only be positive about 50 percent of the time. Cultures, although more reliable, can also yield false-negative results. Accordingly, it is often necessary to repeat such tests several times if the diagnosis is strongly suspected.

Treatment.   Treatment is primarily directed towards eradicating the inflammation by selective administration of antibiotics. Pelvic surgery (other than to remove distended or infected lesions and damaged fallopian tubes) has little therapeutic benefit. Provided that the tuberculous process has not destroyed the uterine lining, IVF following successful antibacterial treatment is the only rational method of treating infertility associated with pelvic tuberculosis.

Endometriosis

Endometriosis is a condition where the endometrium grows on pelvic structures outside the uterine cavity. In early-stage endometriosis there is usually little, if any, visible evidence of anatomical distortion sufficient to compromise ovulation or transportation of the egg from the ovary to the fallopian tube. In contrast, more advanced endometriosis is characterized by the presence of pelvic adhesions sufficient to distort normal pelvic anatomy and interfere with fertilization as well as egg/embryo transportation mechanisms.

Endometriosis often goes unnoticed for many years. Frequently, such women are erroneously said to have so-called unexplained infertility until the diagnosis is finally clinched through direct visualization of the lesions at the time of laparoscopy or laparotomy. Not surprisingly, many patients with unexplained infertility are eventually diagnosed with endometriosis.

Recent medical research has helped shed light on how reproductive problems associated with endometriosis evolve and offers promise with regard to the future treatment of infertility/reproductive failure associated with this condition. One of the most interesting breakthroughs is the finding that endometriosis appears to have a genetic component. In the future, the development of genetic markers might provide an important diagnostic tool.

Grades of severity. In the case of *advanced endometriosis,* inspection at laparoscopy or laparotomy will usually reveal severe pelvic adhesions, scarring, and "chocolate cysts" causally linked to the infertility. The quality of life of women with advanced endometriosis is usually so severely compromised by pain and discomfort that having a baby is often low on the priority list. Accordingly, such patients are usually more interested in relatively radical medical and surgical treatment options that might preclude a subsequent pregnancy, such as removal of ovaries, fallopian tubes, and even the uterus as a means of alleviating suffering. Women with *moderately severe endometriosis* have a modest amount of scarring/adhesions and endometriotic deposits, which are usually detected on the ovaries, fallopian tubes, bladder surface, and low in the pelvis, behind the uterus. In such cases, the fallopian tubes are usually opened and functional. Women with *mild endometriosis* are often erroneously labeled as having unexplained infertility because of the insignificant distortion of pelvic anatomy.

Endometriosis impacts on fertility. To hold that infertility can only be attributed to endometriosis if significant anatomical disease can be identified is to ignore the fact that biochemical, hormonal, and immunological factors profoundly impact fertility. Failure to recognize this salient fact continues to play havoc with the hopes and dreams of many infertile endometriosis patients. The questions that should be asked are why, in the absence of any other apparent cause of infertility,

- women with mild to moderate endometriosis experience a three- to four-fold lower spontaneous conception rate compared to women who do not have endometriosis;
- normally ovulating women with mild to moderate endometriosis do not experience a much-improved pregnancy rate following controlled ovarian hyperstimulation (COH) with clomiphene citrate or gonadotropins, regardless of whether intrauterine insemination (IUI) is done;
- surgery performed on normally ovulating women to remove small endometriotic deposits is unlikely to improve pregnancy rates very much; and
- one-third of women with endometriosis (regardless of severity) have immunologic implantation problems that virtually preclude a viable pregnancy. Such women often fail to conceive even with repeated IVF attempts where numerous good-quality embryos or blastocysts were transferred.

The causes of these problems are toxins in the peritoneal fluid ("the peritoneal factor") and the immunologic rejection of the early embryo as it attempts to implant into the uterine lining. *Toxins* that impair fertilization of the egg are present in the peritoneal secretions of most women who have endometriosis, regardless of its severity. This explains why women with endometriosis are three to four times less likely to conceive per month of trying and why procedures such as intrauterine insemination do not increase the chances of pregnancy. It also explains why IVF, which entails removing eggs through aspiration of the ovarian follicles before they can be affected by peritoneal toxins, improves pregnancy rates dramatically and, accordingly, is the treatment of choice for most endometriosis patients with infertility. (See chapter 8 for a discussion of the role of therapeutic immunomodulation.)

Treatment.   The following basic concepts apply to management of endometriosis-related infertility.

Ovulation induction with or without intrauterine insemination: Because toxins in the peritoneal secretions of women with endometriosis exert a negative effect on fertilization potential regardless of how sperm reaches the fallopian tubes, it follows that intrauterine insemination will not improve the chances of pregnancy much (over no treatment at all) in women with mild to moderate endometriosis.

Surgery: Surgery aimed at restoring the anatomical integrity of the fallopian tubes neither counters the negative influence of toxic peritoneal factors that inherently reduce the chances of conception in women with endometriosis nor addresses the immunologic dysfunction commonly associated with this condition. For this reason, we believe that pelvic surgery is relatively contraindicated for the treatment of infertility associated with endometriosis when the woman is over 35 years old. Impending diminution of ovarian reserve (with premenopause approaching) in such women means that they simply do not have the time to waste on less efficacious alternatives and that IVF is needed. In contrast, younger women with endometriosis, who have time on their side, might consider surgery as a viable option. Approximately 30 to 40 percent of such younger normally ovulating women will conceive within three years following corrective pelvic surgery.

Sclerotherapy of ovarian endometriomas in preparation for IVF: An *endometrioma* is a cystic collection of altered menstrual blood in the ovary that interferes with optimal follicle/egg development such that eggs harvested from the affected ovary are often compromised in their development, yielding poor-quality embryos following IVF. It is for this reason that ovarian endometriomas must be removed prior to ovarian stimulation for IVF. Simple aspiration of endometriomas is unsatisfactory because they will recur. Conventional surgical treatment, which involves either an abdominal incision or laparoscopic drainage of the cyst contents with subsequent removal of the cyst wall, can also be unsatisfactory because, unfortunately, in many cases normal ovarian tissue is inadvertently removed along with the cyst wall, which may decrease the number of eggs available for subsequent fertility treatment. Additionally, visualization of anatomic structures may be obscured by pelvic adhesions, leading to inadequate surgical removal with frequent cyst recurrence and the increased risk of surgical complications. Many patients with recurrent ovarian endometriomas are uncomfortable with the prospect of repeat surgery, and its avoidance is often a factor in the decision to proceed with IVF.

We have performed *sclerotherapy* on more than 200 women with endometriomas who were preparing for treatment with IVF. Sclerotherapy for ovarian endometriomas involves needle aspiration of the liquid content of the endometriotic cyst, followed by the injection of 5 percent tetracycline into the cyst cavity. Treatment results in disappearance of the lesion within six to eight weeks in more than 80 percent of cases so treated. In the remainder, a simple cyst may remain, which in the vast majority of cases resolves permanently following a single aspiration. Ovarian sclerotherapy can be performed under local anesthesia or under general anesthesia. It has the advantage of being a low-cost, ambulatory office-based procedure with a low incidence of significant postprocedural pain or complications and avoidance of the need for laparoscopy or laparotomy. Since sclerotherapy for endometriomas is associated with a small but yet realistic possibility of adhesion formation, it should only be used in cases where IVF is the only treatment available to the patient. Women who intend to try and conceive through fertilization in their fallopian tubes (e.g., following natural conception or intrauterine insemination) will be better off undergoing laparotomy or laparoscopy for the treatment of endometriomas.

In vitro fertilization: IVF is the treatment of choice for women over 35 or where surgery and treatment with fertility agents has proven to be unsuccessful. We anticipate that approximately 75 percent of such women under the age of 40 will achieve the birth of one or more babies within three IVF attempts performed at SIRM.

It is possible and perhaps even likely that women who fit this profile might conceive spontaneously on their own and have a baby in spite of (rather than due to) treatment. Failure to recognize this possibility carries the risk of unjustified complacency brought about by the perception that if a pregnancy occurred with or without treatment, it can be expected to happen just as easily again. Not so. The chances for pregnancy remain three to four times lower than for non-endometriotic, healthy ovulating women of a similar age, whether so treated or not.

While the exact cause of endometriosis remains an enigma, it is now apparent that immunologic dysfunction is a significant feature of this disease. Whether immunopathology is causally linked to this condition or whether it occurs in response to endometriosis is unknown. Regardless, the underlying immunologic disorder adversely impacts on implantation. However, it is possible, by means of thorough and meticulous evaluation, to quantify, typify, and, thereupon, selectively treat the underlying immunopathology. In so doing, IVF pregnancy rates can be significantly improved.

Asherman's Syndrome

Asherman's syndrome is a condition characterized by the presence of severe intrauterine adhesions that often destroy most of the basal layer of the endometrium from which, under the influence of estrogen and progesterone, the endometrium develops. When most of the basal endometrium is incapacitated so that virtually no regeneration of the endometrium can take place, cessation of menstruation and infertility follow.

Asherman's syndrome most commonly results from postpartum or postabortal endometritis; but it can also occur following uterine surgery, such as removal of fibroid tumors that encroach upon or penetrate the uterine cavity.

Treatment involves a procedure called hysteroscopic resection, whereby a telescope-like instrument is introduced via the vagina and cervix into the uterine cavity to allow direct surgical resection of scar tissue. The objective is to remove as much scar tissue as possible and to free adhesions that fuse the walls of the uterine cavity, so as to uncover and enable viable basal endometrium to resume growth and progressively cover as much of the surface of the uterine cavity as possible.

Postoperatively, a small balloon is often placed in the uterine cavity for a day or two to keep the opposing surfaces separated in the hope of preventing recurrence of adhesions. The woman usually receives supplemental estrogen to encourage endometrial growth.

Endometritis severe enough to produce Asherman's syndrome usually scars and blocks the uterine entrance to the fallopian tubes. However, sometimes one or both tubes remain open (although there is usually always some degree of damage to the inner lining). While in such cases the uterus is often incapable of allowing proper embryo implantation, implantation could occur in a fallopian tube, leading to an ectopic pregnancy.

Unfortunately, with Asherman's syndrome there is such widespread destruction of the basal endometrium that improving blood flow with Viagra is often unsuccessful in improving estrogen-mediated endometrial development sufficient to achieve adequate endometrial growth. In such cases, the women should consider stopping all treatment and adopting or attempting gestational surrogacy.

Diethylstilbestrol (DES) and Reproductive Failure

Diethylstilbestrol (DES) was widely prescribed in the late 1950s and early 1960s to try and prevent miscarriages. Today, ectopic pregnancies, miscarriages, premature labor, and both male and female infertility are all relatively prevalent in the offspring of women exposed to DES during the first half of pregnancy (while they were still in their mother's uterus). It is important to recognize, however, that only about 20 percent of women prenatally exposed to DES experience these problems.

DES is a synthetic hormone with profound estrogenlike properties. However, its chemical structure bears no similarity whatsoever to that of natural estrogen. Natural estrogen is a lipid (fatty) substance with a "steroid structure," while DES is a nonlipid chemical containing a "stilbene nucleus." DES is very similar in structure to the fertility agent clomiphene citrate (Serophene, Clomid).

In order for a natural hormone such as estrogen to exert a biological effect, it must first attach to the cell surface at specialized sites called receptors. These receptors are uniquely specific for each hormone.

Paradoxically, DES has great affinity for estrogen receptors and is even capable of displacing estrogen from its own receptor sites.

It is, accordingly, not surprising that the development of reproductive structures such as the upper two thirds of the vagina, cervix, uterus, fallopian tubes in the woman, and sperm ducts in the man, all of which are dependent upon maternal estrogen for their development and which share a common embryologic origin, are adversely influenced by exposure to DES. They are all derived from the Mullerian system, which while initiating development in the first trimester, undergoes maximal development during the second trimester. This could explain why the severity of reproductive abnormalities caused by prenatal DES exposure varies according to the exact time and duration of exposure during the first half of pregnancy. For example, it is highly unlikely that the offspring of women who ingested DES briefly during early pregnancy would have severe developmental abnormalities of the reproductive tract, while the offspring of women who were exposed to DES for an extended period during the third and fourth months of pregnancy would be very likely to be affected.

Fortunately, in the majority of cases DES was usually only prescribed for a brief period of time during the early first trimester of pregnancy while the woman was experiencing vaginal bleeding (a threatened miscarriage) and was discontinued when bleeding stopped. These women usually did not ingest DES during the critical phase of Mullerian development, and the reproductive function of their offspring was left unaffected. That is why only 20 percent of DES-exposed female offspring suffer long-term consequences.

Women who experience reproductive failure due to DES exposure often exhibit characteristic abnormalities of their reproductive tracts. These include structural deformities of the upper vagina and cervix, as well as the presence of glandular tissue (normally absent in the vagina and outer cervix) referred to as vaginal adenosis. The cervical canal, which connects the vagina to the uterine cavity, is often long and distorted in DES-affected women, whose uterine cavities are usually disproportionately short and distorted. Moreover, the walls of the DES uterus tend to be more fibrous, which may result in reduced ability of the uterus to stretch and is responsible for the high incidence of premature births by DES-affected mothers. The abnormal uterine cavity associated with DES exposure can be readily demonstrated through the performance of a hysterosalpingogram, which often reveals a T- or butterfly-shape rather than a normal rounded, pear-shaped appearance.

The fallopian tubes of the DES daughter are also often deformed. They tend to be shorter than normal and have an abnormal inner structure. The typical longitudinal folds of the inner lining of the normal fallopian tube are often absent, irregular, or distorted, a possible explanation for the high ectopic pregnancy rate associated with DES anomalies.

It is important to emphasize that the ovaries are not of Mullerian origin and are, accordingly, unaffected by prenatal DES exposure. DES daughters usually ovulate normally and have normal blood-hormone levels. It is probably for this reason that the cause of reproductive failure sometimes goes undetected in such cases.

The above-mentioned structural abnormalities explain most of the serious reproductive complications that occur in women who were exposed to DES prenatally. However, these anomalies do not completely explain the relatively high incidence of early and recurrent spontaneous miscarriages that so commonly occur in association with DES uterine anomalies. Recent research has demonstrated that prenatal DES exposure at the critical period of Mullerian development might permanently alter the structure and function of estrogen receptors, rendering them permanently incapable of responding appropriately to natural estrogen in later life. This could explain why the endometrium and cervical lining of DES daughters often fail to respond appropriately to estrogen.

Our own research has confirmed that women with obvious Mullerian anomalies secondary to prenatal DES exposure commonly present with cervical mucus insufficiency and a thin endometrial lining in spite of normal blood estrogen concentrations around the time of ovulation. The poor-quality cervical mucus and thin uterine linings might explain the high incidence of infertility associated with DES anomalies. Perhaps the poor thickness and quality of the uterine lining compromises healthy implantation and placentation that is essential for early fetal development and growth.

We believe that the close structural similarity between DES and clomiphene citrate could explain why the administration of clomiphene to DES daughters is more likely to result in an inadequate uterine lining and abnormal quality cervical mucus than in non-DES affected women and probably explains the low pregnancy rate associated with clomiphene therapy in these cases. We have demonstrated in non-DES exposed women that prolonged usage of clomiphene citrate for more than three consecutive months almost invariably results in progressive and often profound thinning of the endometrium as well as cervical mucus insufficiency, thereby producing a relative "contraceptive effect." We have further observed that this tendency is far more profound when clomiphene is administered to women with DES Mullerian anomalies and, accordingly, rarely recommend the administration of clomiphene citrate in such cases.

And so it is that ill-conceived administration of DES to women over 40 years ago, without clear evidence of potential benefit, resulted in serious reproductive consequences to their offspring. Perhaps we will learn an important lesson from this tragedy, one that calls upon the medical profession to resist the temptation of administering medications to patients simply on anecdotal grounds. We should insist upon evidence of benefit before recommending the administration of untried therapeutic regimens if we are to avoid a repetition of the DES disaster.

The thin uterine lining associated with DES uterine abnormalities is often successfully treated with vaginal Viagra suppositories. In fact, the first woman ever to conceive with IVF following such treatment had experienced a restoration of her uterine lining with vaginal Viagra therapy.

Ectopic Pregnancy

By definition, an ectopic pregnancy is a gestation that occurs outside of the uterine cavity. The most common site is in the fallopian tube, but sometimes it can occur in the ovary, the cervix, or even the abdominal cavity. Ectopic pregnancy is one of the most dangerous complications of pregnancy. If undetected, the ectopic pregnancy will continue to grow and will ultimately burst through the wall of the fallopian tube, often resulting in catastrophic intra-abdominal bleeding, which can be fatal.

Estimates put the incidence of ectopic pregnancy at about one in 200 pregnancies, but it has been reported to occur in about one out of 30 pregnancies resulting from IVF. A woman who has had one ectopic pregnancy has almost four times as great a risk of an ectopic in a future pregnancy, and with every subsequent ectopic this risk increases dramatically.

The introduction of sophisticated sonographic and hormonal-monitoring technology now makes it possible to detect an ectopic pregnancy very early on, well in advance of its rupturing. A decade or two ago, the diagnosis of an ectopic pregnancy, ruptured or not, was an indication for immediate laparotomy (a wide incision made in the abdominal wall) to avoid the risk of catastrophic hemorrhagic shock. This often resulted in complete removal of the affected fallopian tube, sometimes along with the adjacent ovary.

In the late 1980s, conservative early surgical intervention by laparoscopy began replacing laparotomy for the treatment of ectopic pregnancy, often allowing the affected fallopian tube to be preserved and shortening the period of postsurgical convalescence. In the 1990s, early detection combined with the advent of medical management with methotrexate (MTX) has all but eliminated the need for surgical intervention in the majority of patients (see below).

Causes of ectopic pregnancy. Because fertilization of the human egg normally takes place in the fallopian tube, anything that delays the passage of the embryo down the fallopian tube into the uterus can result in the embryo hatching, sending its root system into the wall of the fallopian tube and initiating growth within the tube. One of the most common predisposing factors for ectopic pregnancy is PID, which damages the *endosalpinx* (inner lining of the fallopian tubes). The endosalpinx has a very complex and delicate internal architecture, with small hairs and secretions that help to propel the embryo toward the uterine cavity, and once damaged by PID can never regenerate completely. This is one of the reasons why women who manage to conceive following surgery to unblock fallopian tubes damaged by

PID have about a one in four chance of developing a subsequent ectopic pregnancy.

Congenital malformations of the fallopian tube, associated with shortening of or small pockets and side channels within the tube that can interrupt the smooth passage of the embryo down the tube, are another cause of an ectopic pregnancy.

Since the lining of the fallopian tube does not represent an optimal site for healthy implantation, a large percentage of pregnancies that gain early attachment to its inner lining will likely be absorbed before the woman even knows that she is pregnant. This is often referred to as a *tubal abortion.*

Symptoms of ectopic pregnancy. The classical picture of ectopic pregnancy include the following symptoms:

1. Missed menstrual period, as in early pregnancy, although some patients will have spotting or other abnormal bleeding. The pregnancy test will be positive in such cases.

2. Pain, typically cramplike in nature, located on one or another side of the lower abdomen, caused by spasm of the muscular wall of the fallopian tube(s). In cases where the ectopic pregnancy has ruptured and bleeding has occurred into the abdominal cavity, the woman often experiences severe abdominal pain that increases progressively in severity and is worse on movement. This is because blood irritates the peritoneal membrane, which envelops all abdominal-pelvic organs. Sometimes the woman will experience pain in the right shoulder because blood that tracks along the side of the abdominal cavity finds its way to the area immediately below the diaphragm, above the liver (on the woman's right side), and irritates the endings of the phrenic nerve, which supplies that part of the diaphragm. This results in the referral of the pain to the neck and shoulder.

3. Vaginal bleeding. When a pregnancy inadvertently implants in the fallopian tube, the lining of the uterus undergoes profound hormonal changes associated with pregnancy (primarily associated with the hormone progesterone). When the embryo dies, the lining of the uterus separates from the uterine wall. Initially, vaginal bleeding is dark and usually is quite scanty, even less than with a normal menstrual period. In some cases of ectopic pregnancy, bleeding is more severe, similar to that experienced in association with a miscarriage. This sometimes leads to ectopic pregnancy initially being misdiagnosed as a miscarriage and is the reason for the need to examine the material that is passed vaginally for evidence of products of conception.

4. Dizziness and/or fainting. This is usually a late symptom, indicative of tubal rupture, internal bleeding, and impending shock. It is an indication to seek *immediate* medical attention.

Diagnosis of ectopic pregnancy. The easiest and most common method of diagnosing an ectopic pregnancy is by tracking the rate of rise in the blood levels of the "hormone of pregnancy," hCG. With a normal intrauterine pregnancy, blood levels of hCG will usually double every two days throughout the first nine to ten weeks. While an inappropriate rate of increase in hCG usually suggests an impending miscarriage, it might also point to an ectopic pregnancy. Thus the hCG levels should be followed serially until a clear pattern emerges.

The diagnosis of an ectopic pregnancy is often clinched by ultrasound examination, which is performed using a sensitive ultrasound machine. Given sufficient expertise, this will often reveal an unruptured ectopic pregnancy within a fallopian tube. If the tube has already ruptured or internal bleeding has occurred, ultrasound examination will inevitably detect the presence of free fluid into the abdominal cavity.

If there has been a significant amount of intra-abdominal bleeding, irritation of the peritoneal membrane will cause the abdominal wall to become tense and, depending on the amount of blood in the abdomen, to distend. In such cases, any pressure on the abdominal wall will evoke significant pain; and when a vaginal examination is done, movement of the cervix produces excruciating pain, especially on the side of the affected fallopian tube.

Typical presentation of a ruptured ectopic pregnancy. When a tubal ectopic pregnancy ruptures it represents an abdominal catastrophe. The woman will often collapse with severe pain. She will be in shock, pale, have a rapid pulse with a low blood pressure, and will often be breathing rapidly with demonstrable "air hunger." The clinical picture is often so typical that in most cases, the diagnosis will present no difficulty at all.

Differential diagnosis.   The most important conditions to differentiate from an ectopic pregnancy are (1) a hemorrhagic or a ruptured cyst of the ovary, (2) appendicitis, (3) acute PID, and (4) an inevitable miscarriage.

Surgical management of ectopic pregnancy.   In questionable situations, laparoscopy is usually performed for diagnostic purposes. If an ectopic pregnancy is in fact detected, a small longitudinal incision over the tubal pregnancy (*linear salpingectomy*) will allow its removal without necessitating removal of the tube. Bleeding points on the fallopian tube can usually be accessed directly and appropriately ligated through the laparoscope. Sometimes the damage to the fallopian tube has been so extensive that the entire tube will require removal.

On occasions where very severe intra-abdominal bleeding heralds a potential catastrophe, a laparotomy (an incision made to open the abdominal cavity) is immediately performed to stop the bleeding. In such cases, a blood transfusion is usually required and may be life-saving.

Medical management of ectopic pregnancy.   The introduction of methotrexate (MTX) therapy for the treatment of ectopic pregnancy has profoundly reduced the need for surgery in most patients. MTX is a chemotherapeutic that kills rapidly dividing cells, such as those present in the root system of the conceptus. Extremely low doses of MTX are used to treat ectopic pregnancy. Accordingly, the side effects that are often associated with such chemotherapy used for the treatment of other conditions are seldom seen. It is important to confirm that the ectopic pregnancy has not yet ruptured prior to administering MTX.

The administration of MTX is by intramuscular injection. Prior to its administration, blood is drawn to get a baseline blood hCG level. After the injection of MTX, the woman is allowed to return home with strict instructions that she should always have someone with her and never be alone in the ensuing week. The concern is that were the patient to be on her own and an intra-abdominal bleed were to occur, she might not readily be able to access someone who could get her to the hospital immediately. Instructions are also given to look for early signs that might point towards severe intra-abdominal bleeding, such as the sudden onset of severe pain, light-headedness, or fainting.

The patient returns to the doctor's office about four days later to check the blood hCG level. Thereupon, in three days (seven days after MTX) the level is checked again. By this time the hCG level should have dropped at about 50 percent from the value on day 4. If not, a second MTX injection is given, and the blood levels are tested twice weekly until the hCG level is undetectable. Once this occurs, vaginal bleeding will usually ensue within a week or two.

It is important to note, especially in cases where more than one embryo or blastocyst has been transferred to the uterine cavity or fallopian tube (see chapter 13, "Zygote Intrafallopian Transfer or Tubal Embryo Transfer"), that implantation may occur in two sites simultaneously (i.e., in the fallopian tube as well as inside the uterine cavity). This is referred to as a *heterotopic pregnancy*. It is therefore important that before administering MTX, which will cause the death and absorption of any early pregnancy, it must be determined that the physician is not dealing with a heterotopic pregnancy. In the case of a heterotopic pregnancy, surgery is required to treat the tubal ectopic pregnancy while every precaution is taken to protect the pregnancy growing within the uterine cavity.

Thrombophilias

Thrombophilia is the inherited tendency to develop blood clots too easily. Thrombophilias are due either to the presence of too much of certain blood-clotting factors or too little of anti-clotting proteins in the blood. As many as one in five people in the United States has a thrombophilia.

Most women with a thrombophilia have healthy pregnancies. However, thrombophilias can contribute to a number of pregnancy complications, including pregnancy loss in the second or third trimester (i.e., stillbirths), placental abruption (when the placenta separates from the uterine wall, partially or completely, before delivery), and poor fetal growth. The thrombophilias are also associated with an increased risk of preeclampsia, (a pregnancy-related disorder characterized by high blood pressure and protein in the urine that can pose serious risks for mother and baby). Several of these problems are believed to result from blood clots in placental blood vessels that lead to changes in the placenta and reduced blood flow to the fetus. In the postpartum period, women with thrombophilias will have an increased risk of developing deep-vein thrombosis and pulmonary embolus.

Pregnant women in general are more likely than nonpregnant women to develop a venous thrombotic episode (VTE), or development of a blood clot in a vein. This is due to normal pregnancy-related changes in blood clotting in order to limit blood loss during labor and delivery. And pregnant women with a thrombophilia are at a higher risk than other pregnant women of developing a VTE. Studies suggest that more than half of pregnant women who develop a VTE have an underlying thrombophilia.

All pregnant women who have had a blood clot should be offered testing for hereditary thrombophilias. In addition, women with a family history of blood clots, pulmonary embolism (blood clot in the lung), strokes that occurred prior to age 60, or a history of pregnancy complications, including stillbirth, early or severe preeclampsia, placental abruption, or poor fetal growth due to undetermined causes, may be considered for testing.

Some pregnant women with a thrombophilia are treated with high doses of folic acid and others in addition may require one or more daily injections of low-dose heparin, a blood-thinning drug that does not cross the placenta and is safe for the baby.

Not all pregnant women with a thrombophilia need twice daily heparin treatment during pregnancy. Regular heparin can be supplanted with a newer form of heparin called low-molecular-weight heparin, which appears to pose a lower risk of side effects such as bone loss and can be injected once instead of twice daily (as with regular heparin) and which significantly reduces the risk of local bruising.

Warfarin (also a blood-thinning drug) may be used safely in addition to, or instead of, heparin in the postpartum period and during breast feeding. However, it is not recommended during pregnancy because it can cause birth defects.

Presently no proven cause-and-effect relationship has been shown to exist between thrombophilia on the one hand and failed embryo implantation, poor IVF outcome, and/or early recurrent miscarriages on the other.

Polycystic Ovarian Syndrome (PCOS)

Polycystic ovarian syndrome (PCOS) occurs in 5–10 percent of women of reproductive age. The condition is characterized by abnormal ovarian function (irregular or absent periods, abnormal or absent ovulation, and infertility); increased body hair; acne; and increased body weight. It is also often associated with insulin-resistant high blood insulin levels and non-insulin-dependent diabetes mellitus, which contribute to the development of obesity, an abnormal lipid profile, and cardiovascular disease. Women with PCOS are also at slightly increased risk of developing uterine, ovarian, and possibly also breast cancer and accordingly should be evaluated carefully on an annual or more frequent basis.

PCOS-related infertility is usually manageable through selective surgery and/or the use of oral and/or injectable fertility drugs.

There are three basic forms of PCOS:

1. **Hypothalamic-pituitary-ovarian:** This, the most common form of PCOS, is often genetically transmitted. It is characteristically associated with an LH concentration in the blood that is higher than the FSH level (usually, the opposite is the case), as well as high concentrations of androgens (male hormones) and resistance to insulin. Ovulation induction with fertility drugs such as clomiphene citrate, Letrozole, or gonadotropins, with or without IUI, is often highly successful in establishing pregnancies in women with PCOS. However, IVF is fast becoming a treatment of choice. In about 40 percent of cases, three to six months of oral Metformin treatment results in a significant improvement. Surgical treatment by "ovarian drilling" of the many small ovarian cysts lying immediately below the capsule of the ovaries is often used but is less successful than non-surgical treatment and is only temporarily effective.

2. **Adrenal:** Androgens are also raised here, as is the level of dehydroepriandrosterone (DHEAS), which confirms the adrenal origin of

this androgen. Adrenal PCOS is treated with steroids, which over a period of several weeks will suppress adrenal androgen production, allowing regular ovulation to take place spontaneously.

3. Severe pelvic adhesive disease secondary to severe endometriosis, chronic PID, and extensive pelvic surgery: Women who have this type of PCOS tend to be much less responsive to stimulation with gonadotropins, and androgen levels may vary. DHEAS is not raised.

IVF is becoming the primary and preferential treatment for PCOS because it is only through IVF that the number of embryos reaching the uterus can be controlled and the risk of high-order multiple pregnancies can be minimized. In addition, only in the course of IVF treatment can prolonged coasting, which prevents OHSS, be implemented (see later in this section).

Women with PCOS are at an inordinate risk of severely overresponding to gonadotropin fertility drugs such as Repronex, Follistim, and/or Bravelle with the formation of large numbers (often over 25) ovarian follicles. They also often experience multiple ovulations, which dramatically increases the risk of multiple pregnancy (40 to 50 percent), often resulting in high-order multiple gestations. In addition, the overstimulation with gonadotropins can be so severe as to become life-endangering (e.g., severe ovarian hyperstimulation syndrome [OHSS]).

Severe ovarian hyperstimulation syndrome (OHSS). The onset of OHSS is signaled by the development of a large number of ovarian follicles (usually more than 25), accompanied by rapidly rising blood estradiol. Symptoms include abdominal distention due to fluid collection, fluid in the chest cavity, rapid weight gain due to tissue fluid retention, abdominal pain, lower back ache, nausea, diarrhea, vomiting, visual disturbances, a rapidly declining urine output, cardiovascular collapse, and failure of blood to clot. These signs may occur before pregnancy can be diagnosed. If pregnancy occurs, the condition is likely to worsen progressively over a period of three to five weeks, whereupon it rapidly resolves spontaneously over a few days. If no pregnancy occurs, the symptoms and signs all disappear spontaneous-ly within 10 to 12 days of the hCG injection.

When increasing fluid collection in the abdominal cavity starts to compromise breathing, raising the head of the bed slightly by placing a four- to six-inch block at the base of each head post and using addi-tional pillows will sometimes help ameliorate the problem. In cases where this does not help or symptoms become severe, all or most of the fluid can safely be drained by transvaginal sterile-needle aspiration once or twice weekly. The problem usually corrects itself within 10 to 12 days of the hCG shot if pregnancy does not occur, or by the eighth week of pregnancy.

Urine output should be monitored daily to see if it drops below 500 ml a day. A chest X-ray to evaluate for fluid collection in the chest and around the heart should be done weekly along with a battery of blood tests. In case of a deteriorating clinical situation, hospitalization might be needed for close observation and, if necessary, to provide for inten-sive care.

In all cases of OHSS, the ovaries will invariably be considerably enlarged. This is irrelevant to the final outcome unless the twist of the ovary on its axis, an extremely rare complication, occurs. This would usually require emergency surgical intervention.

It is important to know that symptoms and signs of OHSS are severely aggravated by rising hCG levels. Thus, women with OHSS should not receive additional hCG injections.

Does PCOS cause poor egg/embryo quality?   Women with PCOS undergoing IVF are commonly found to have poorly developed eggs with reduced potential for fertilization and yielding poor-quality embryos. However, it is unlikely to be due to an intrinsic deficit in egg quality; rather, it more likely relates to intra-ovarian hormonal changes brought about by hyperstimulation. This effect can often be signifi-cantly reduced through implementation of an individualized ovarian stimulation protocol that minimizes exposure of the developing folli-cles and eggs to excessive LH-induced ovarian androgens. This can best be achieved by limiting the use of LH-containing gonadotropins such as Repronex and through selective institution of prolonged coasting.

In the past, the onset of OHSS, heralded by the presence of large numbers of developing ovarian follicles and rapidly rising plasma estradiol levels, often led the treating physician to prematurely administer hCG in an attempt to abruptly arrest the process and prevent escalation of risk to the patient. However, the premature administration of hCG, while abruptly arresting further proliferation of estrogen-producing granulose cells in the follicles, unfortunately also prematurely arrests egg development. Since the ability of an egg to achieve optimal maturation upon hCG triggering is largely predicated upon its having achieved optimal development, the untimely administration of hCG, which triggers meiosis, probably increases the risk of chromosome abnormalities of the egg. This, in turn, would lead to reduced fertilization potential, poor egg/embryo quality, and low potential for embryo implantation.

While excessive exposure of developing eggs to ovarian androgens compromises follicle and egg growth, it also impairs endometrial response to estrogen, which could explain the common finding of poor endometrial thickening in many women with PCOS undergoing IVF.

The obvious remedy for these adverse effects on egg and endometrial development is to employ stimulation protocols that limit ovarian overexposure to LH and allow the time necessary for the follicles/eggs to develop optimally prior to administering hCG through the judicious implementation of prolonged coasting.

Prolonged coasting.   In the early 1990s we were the first to report on prolonged coasting, a novel approach that protects egg quality while preventing the development of OHSS. Prolonged coasting has since gained widespread acceptance as a method of choice for preventing OHSS and has established itself as the standard of care. It involves withholding gonadotropin therapy while continuing the administration of the GnRHa and waiting until the blood estradiol concentration drops below 3000 pg/ml, when hCG is administered. In such cases, regardless of the number of developed follicles or number of eggs retrieved, the woman rarely, if ever, develops OHSS.

The precise timing of prolonged coasting is critical. When initiated too early, follicle growth and development may cease; when started too late, the follicles will harbor malformed eggs.

COMPARING APPLES AND ORANGES—TUBAL SURGERY VS. IVF

Blockage of the fallopian tubes is one of the most common causes of infertility. As explained earlier in this chapter, tubal damage is often caused by PID, endometriosis, previous abdominal surgery (especially due to a ruptured appendix or ruptured ovarian cyst), and ectopic pregnancy.

Even if procedures such as laparoscopy or HSG determine that the tubes are patent, with a history of PID there is likely to be damage within the tube that destroys its normal functions. PID is one of the most common causes of tubal damage that almost always affects both tubes, and even if one tube is open it is still highly likely to be functionally compromised. While surgery can open tubes, it cannot restore normal function. Tubal disease, especially if it is due to PID, is best treated by IVF.

In the case of hydrosalpynx (the fallopian tubes are distended with fluid), tubes so affected must be ligated at the junction with the uterus or removed lest they compromise IVF outcome. Removal (salpingectomy) is preferable to ligation because it is the only sure way to avert pain and complications in the long run.

In our opinion, given the high success rates with IVF performed in good programs, surgery to repair damaged tubes, with few exceptions, can no longer be justified financially or ethically. Other than *tubal reanastomosis* (surgical reconnection of the fallopian tubes, usually performed after a previous tubal ligation), the only time that tubal surgery would occasionally enhance the ability to conceive is when the fimbriated ends of the fallopian tubes are normal. Without functional fimbriae, it is highly unlikely that an egg would find its way from the ovary into the fallopian tube. For example, surgically reopening the end of a blocked fallopian tube (often eliminating the fimbriae) provides relatively little hope for the infertile couple. In such cases, the woman often stands less than a 20 percent chance of having a baby within two years of tubal surgery, whereas the same woman would have better than a 40 percent chance after a single attempt at IVF performed in an optimal IVF program. In addition, such major surgery carries with it prolonged hospitalization, the risk

of complications, increased cost, and lost time away from work, inca-
pacitation, and significantly greater discomfort.

A reasonable birthrate of about 40 percent can be expected within
two to three years of reproductive surgery to remove adhesions surrounding the fallopian tubes as long as the fimbriae and the insides of
the tubes are otherwise normal. Women under 35 under such circumstances still may choose surgery over IVF in such cases, provided they
are willing to allow two to three years for the surgery to have a good
chance to work. It is, however, a reality that more than 70 percent of
women who undergo tubal surgery for the treatment of infertility will
ultimately require IVF.

As long as insurance companies in the United States reimburse for
about 80 percent of the costs of tubal surgery but are unwilling to fund
IVF, and as long as consumers remain uninformed about the benefits
of IVF, most couples will still select tubal surgery over IVF for financial
reasons. Two-thirds of all tubal surgeries performed in the United
States are still being done in cases where for all practical purposes the
fallopian tubes have been irreparably damaged. In the remaining one-
third, tubal surgery is more appropriately performed to free adhesions
around the fallopian tubes and ovaries, remove fibroid tumors, and
treat endometriosis.

Actually, comparing tubal surgery with IVF is a futile exercise. How
can a procedure such as IVF, where success rates are determined on
the basis of a single menstrual cycle of treatment, be compared with
tubal surgery, in which evaluation of the success rate per procedure
requires a wait-and-see approach that often spans two or more years?
Three or four attempts at IVF, performed even in the average IVF setting, are likely to result in a higher success rate than any form of tubal
surgery.

The insurance environment surrounding IVF in the United States
can be expected to ultimately change if current legislative and judicial
trends continue (see chapter 15). As more lawmakers and courts direct
insurance carriers to fund IVF, the popularity of IVF will inevitably
surpass that of most forms of tubal surgery. We predict that when the
financial burden is eliminated, virtually all women would choose IVF
in preference to undergoing major tubal surgery.

Table 9-1
TUBAL SURGERY VS. IVF

	Tubal Surgery	*IVF*
Risk of complications	+	−
Cost (out-of-pocket)	+	++
Risk of ectopic pregnancy	++	+

+ = moderate
− = almost absent
++ = great

In general, the forms of sterilization that can best be reversed microsurgically are those in which a small portion of the fallopian tube was either blocked or cut away at one place in the mid-portion of the tube. In such cases, there is a 70 to 80 percent chance that patency (absence of blockage) of at least one fallopian tube can be reestablished successfully through tubal reconstructive surgery. The subsequent birthrate is approximately 50 percent within three years after the procedure. Restoration of tubal patency after sterilization gives the woman a permanent chance of conceiving. Therefore, this is one of the few situations in which we might recommend tubal surgery over IVF—provided the woman undergoing the procedure is under 35.

It should also be recognized, however, that a single cycle of IVF performed in the optimal setting could afford the same woman at least the same chance of having a baby from a single attempt, provided tubal occlusion was the only reason for her infertility problem. Two IVF attempts in an optimal setting would almost certainly result in pregnancy rates that surpass those that could be obtained through the performance of tubal reconnection. Moreover, if such a woman desired to retain her contraceptive ability after IVF has produced a baby, her fallopian tubes would still be occluded and her contraception intact. In contrast, following tubal reanastomosis, the woman will have to use some form of contraception.

Another point to be considered is that a 3 percent tubal or ectopic pregnancy rate occurs following IVF pregnancy, as compared with approximately a 15 to 20 percent risk following the performance of tubal reanastomosis.

It is advisable that the opportunities offered by both tubal reanastomosis and IVF be carefully discussed with the couple so they can make
an informed decision. The reason for the relatively high success rates
following tubal reanastomosis is that aside from a small segment of the
fallopian tube that is surgically occluded at the time of sterilization
(and is removed when reanastomosis is performed), the remainder of
the tube is almost always normal. In contrast, the fallopian tubes are
damaged to a lesser or greater degree through disease in almost all
other cases where tubal surgery is performed. This explains the difference in success rates referred to in this section.

CHAPTER

10

IS IVF THE
MOST APPROPRIATE
OPTION?

No couple should attempt IVF until they are certain that no other method of treating infertility would be more appropriate for their particular situation. Since the cause of a problem determines its solution, the couple must first identify the cause of their infertility in order to determine whether they are good candidates for IVF.

Accordingly, a physician with expertise in infertility should examine and evaluate them. The physician will perform certain baseline tests on both partners, and within a month or two should be able to diagnose the problem and prescribe treatment. (As explained in chapter 3, infertility may be caused by either the woman or the man, or both partners may contribute to some degree.) If the cause cannot be pinpointed, the physician might recommend IVF as a means to help diagnose and/or treat infertility.

WHEN IS THE MAN READY FOR IVF?

Evaluation of male fertility revolves around assessing the quality of the sperm, which must be thoroughly evaluated by all possible methods before the couple resort to IVF. This interactive process, which requires cooperation among the urologist, the reproductive endocrinologist or gynecologist, the laboratory, and the couple, has three stages: (1) The urologist seeks specific causes for poor semen quality so therapy can be directed at improving it, (2) the laboratory performs tests that evaluate sperm function and often can enhance the sperms' ability to fertilize an egg, and (3) IVF/ICSI can be used if necessary to achieve fertilization.

Male infertility can be treated by surgically repairing anatomical defects in the reproductive tract or by administering hormones to stimulate the testicles. In rare situations, a disease outside the reproductive tract that hinders sperm production may be corrected medically or surgically. In other cases, there may be very severe structural problems within the sperm ducts brought about by infection, trauma, or even surgery, such as a vasectomy. In cases of total absence of sperm production due to improperly developed testes, usually very little can be done to improve male fertility. When the sperm ducts are blocked, surgical methods can sometimes restore patency; but this does not necessarily mean even if the man can subsequently produce an adequate amount of sperm that he will be able to initiate pregnancy. If the cause of the man's infertility is not correctable through minor surgery or administration of hormones, IVF/ICSI becomes the option of choice.

The probability of successful fertilization occurring either within the petri dish or within the fallopian tube is lower when male-factor infertility is present because as the total number of normal, motile sperm decreases, the fertilization rate also declines. However, the introduction of ICSI has changed all that. Without question, ICSI has made IVF the treatment of choice for moderate or severe male infertility that is unresponsive to simple medical or surgical correction. Now it is possible to achieve the same fertilization and birthrates in cases of male infertility as with indications for IVF. Furthermore, even men who produce no sperm at all in their ejaculates can produce sperm by means of testicular sperm extraction (TESE) or testicular sperm aspiration (TESA), followed by ICSI on their partner's eggs, and still father their own children.

We state categorically that because of dismal success rates in cases of moderate or severe male infertility, intrauterine insemination (IUI) is inadvisable in such cases. The performance of gamete intrafallopian transfer (GIFT) is also relatively contraindicated in cases of male infertility because while GIFT might provide a chance of pregnancy occurring, it is much less effective than IVF/ICSI.

Many of the tests that the male partner of a couple considering IVF should undergo for the purpose of assessment and possible treatment of sperm function are discussed below.

Semen Analysis

The sperm's morphology (percentage of normally shaped sperm), configuration, motility (ability to travel through the reproductive tract and fertilize an egg), and count (number produced in a semen specimen) can be determined under the laboratory microscope in a standard semen analysis or, as is now much more commonly the case, by computerized evaluation. Sperm that appear to be normally shaped are more likely to fertilize an egg, while those with obvious structural abnormalities are less likely or perhaps cannot do so at all. Sophisticated testing may be necessary if the problem cannot be readily identified. However, it is possible for the man to be fertile even when the percentage of normal sperm is low.

Varicocele

The urologist looks for anatomical abnormalities, evidence of obstruction in the scrotum, and physical signs of infection. One anatomical abnormality would be a varicocele, an enlargement of veins in the scrotum, which results in elevated temperatures around the testes that may harm sperm production. In carefully selected cases, tying off or occluding these veins under X-ray visualization may improve semen quality.

Obstruction of the Vas Deferens or Epididymis

When the sperm count is zero and the FSH is normal, the cause may be due to obstruction of the vas deferens or epididymis. If so, TESE/TESA addresses the problem.

Hormonal Problems

If the sperm count or motility initially appear to be abnormal, the physician should determine whether hormonal problems are the cause. This might require extensive blood testing to evaluate the function of the thyroid gland, the output of the pituitary gland, and the secretion of sex hormones by the testicles into the man's blood. In cases of absent sperm in the ejaculate (azoospermia), measurement of blood FSH levels will usually permit distinguishing between testicular failure and obstruction of sperm ducts. If the FSH is elevated, it points to the former, while if the FSH is normal, it is suggestive of the latter (i.e., obstruction). Similarly, in cases of oligozoospermia (low sperm count), the detection of an elevated FSH suggests intractable testicular failure, while a low FSH level is suggestive of potentially reversible (using clomiphene gonadotropins) under-production of sperm by the testes.

The Zona-Free Hamster-Egg Penetration Test (Sperm Penetration Assay, SPA)

A technique known as the zona-free hamster-egg penetration test helps determine whether the sperm are likely to fertilize healthy eggs. In this test, the sperm are placed in a laboratory dish along with hamster eggs from which the eggshell-like zona pellucida has been removed. Then the number of sperm that penetrate the eggs are counted and evaluated. Failure to penetrate a sufficient percentage of eggs may indicate severe male infertility. (Although hamster eggs can be penetrated by human sperm, they will not cleave and develop into viable embryos.)

One of the drawbacks of the zona-free hamster-egg penetration test is that it may produce misleading results. For example, a small percentage of women whose partners failed the hamster test subsequently get pregnant. In other cases, the test results will appear to be normal although the man's fertility is severely impaired. Because this test has a high potential for error, various laboratories may interpret it differently, with conflicting results.

The Hemi-Zona Test

The hemi-zona test uses eggs from surgically removed ovaries or human cadavers. Prior to the test, the eggs are rendered unfertilizable by bisecting them or aspirating their contents; they are then exposed to sperm. By observing the sperm interaction with the eggs, laboratory personnel are able to determine whether the sperm are capable of attaching to or penetrating the surface of the eggs and, thus, whether the acrosome reaction can take place. The hemi-zona test augments but does not replace the zona-free hamster-egg penetration test as a screening method for male-factor infertility. Moreover, the availability of cadaver eggs limits the feasibility of this test.

Testicular Sperm Extraction (TESE) or Testicular Sperm Aspiration (TESA)

TESE/TESA enables men with sperm duct blockage due to trauma, inflammation, a previous vasectomy, or *azoospermia* (no sperm in the ejaculate due to poor testicular sperm production) to father a child through IVF almost as if there were no obstruction to sperm passage at all. The procedures have rendered surgical vasectomy reversal in men with long-standing vasectomies (10 years or more) totally unnecessary. TESE/TESA are both simple, low-cost, safe, and relatively pain-free. Most men can literally take off a few hours for the procedure and return to normal activity soon thereafter. And unlike vasectomy reversal, the procedure allows the man to retain his vasectomy for future contraception purposes.

TESE involves the introduction of a needle through the skin of the scrotum directly into the testicle(s), a 15- to 30-minute procedure usually under local anesthesia. Hair-thin specimens of testicular tissue are removed, sperm is extracted from the tissue, and a single sperm is injected into each egg using ICSI. TESA involves direct aspiration of sperm via the needle inserted into a sperm duct. Following successful TESE/TESA the fertilization rate is 70 percent when ICSI is performed in centers of excellence. The IVF birthrate per TESE procedure performed on women under 40 in these centers is better than 40 percent (i.e., no different than conventional IVF birthrates in women of comparable age). When TESE is performed on men with azoospermia, pregnancy rates are halved.

Microsurgical Epididymal Aspiration (MESA)

MESA involves making an incision in the scrotum and exposing the small sperm-collecting ducts on the surface of the testicles. Sperm is aspirated through a needle inserted into these ducts. The method is much more traumatic and invasive than are either TESE or TESA and only has a place in cases where it is intended to collect enough sperm to perform IVF/ICI with some sperm left over for freezing.

An Abnormal SDIA

An abnormal SDIA (see chapter 8) augers poorly for but does not totally preclude a successful IVF/ICSI pregnancy. However, the prognosis worsens progressively as the age of the egg provider advances beyond 35 years. Selective surgical or medical treatment can sometimes cause the SDIA to revert to normal, such as antioxidant therapy taken for 10 to 12 weeks. Men who have varicoceles associated with an abnormal SDIA may experience a reversion of the SDIA to normal from three to six months following surgical or radiological excision of the varicocele. In rare cases, abnormal SDIA results revert to normal spontaneously. Upon reversion of the SDIA to normal, sperm is collected and cryopreserved for later use. If, in spite of treatment (which presently should be regarded as being in the experimental realm) a grossly abnormal SDIA fails to revert to normal, the use of donor sperm becomes an option, especially where the egg provider is over 35.

WHEN IS THE WOMAN READY FOR IVF?

As in the man's case, defining the cause of a woman's infertility requires careful analysis of her history and a clinical examination by a fertility specialist. Three areas need to be carefully assessed: (1) the pattern of ovulation, (2) the anatomical integrity of the reproductive tract, and (3) the status of the cervical mucus.

The Pattern of Ovulation

As explained in chapter 2, a woman is unlikely to conceive unless she ovulates at the right time in the proper hormonal environment. Reliable evidence of ovulation can only be obtained by examining the woman's ovaries through a laparoscope, by repeated ultrasound examinations around the time of presumed ovulation (to detect a collapsed follicle and/or some follicular fluid pooled in the abdominal cavity), or—the only really reliable way—by confirming a pregnancy with ultrasound.

It is important to remember that the purpose of assessing ovulation is not simply to determine whether the woman ovulated but whether she ovulated at the proper time, within the proper hormonal setting, and if the lining of the uterus is properly prepared. While the following tests will not provide conclusive evidence that the woman has ovulated, they will help the physician determine how well synchronized these vital components are during the luteal phase (second half) of the menstrual cycle. These tests are valuable indicators of the appropriateness of ovulation and the hormonal environment when their results are considered together.

The BBT chart. One way to assess the pattern of ovulation is by compiling a daily body temperature chart. The woman does this by taking her oral temperature each morning before she gets out of bed and before she has anything to drink. She then charts her temperature on a *basal body temperature* (BBT) chart. The pattern on the chart will mirror the output of the hormone progesterone by the corpus luteum in the ovary. A woman's temperature begins rising about 12 to 24 hours following ovulation, and this rise will be sustained through the rest of the menstrual cycle (when the ovaries are producing hormones to prepare the endometrium). In other words, the woman's temperature goes up when progesterone is produced and stays up until its levels drop with the demise of the corpus luteum. This phenomenon occurs because progesterone acts on the biological thermostat in the brain that regulates body temperature, setting it one notch higher when progesterone is being produced and lowering it at or just before the beginning of the menstrual period. As long as the temperature is up, it can be assumed that progesterone is present.

Because ovulation usually occurs 14 days before the expected menstrual period, the woman's temperature will usually be about 0.5°–1°F higher during the last two weeks of her cycle. A biphasic pattern such as this (the first phase is lower than the second phase) suggests ovulation. It is not important whether the increase is sudden or gradual.

Figure 10-1 shows how the biphasic BBT pattern is synchronized with hormone production, ovulation, and other aspects of the menstrual cycle. Estrogen levels in the blood (including estradiol, as shown in figure 10-1) peak at the time of ovulation. This triggers the LH surge and to a lesser extent a synchronous rapid rise and fall in the FSH levels. The woman ovulates eight to 36 hours after LH is first detected in the urine by home ovulation testing. About a day later the temperature rises. The estrogen level falls progressively immediately prior to and for a few hours following ovulation and then rises again, only to drop precipitously immediately prior to menstruation. Measurable amounts of progesterone first appear in the bloodstream around the time of ovulation and then escalate during the second half of the menstrual cycle and, as with estrogen levels, also drop sharply preceding the onset of menstruation.

All of these hormonal interrelationships are orchestrated by the follicle, which contains the developing egg and produces estrogen. Immediately after ovulation, the follicle collapses and forms the corpus luteum, which during the second half of the menstrual cycle produces both estrogen and progesterone. The corpus luteum has a natural life span of about 12 to 14 days, whereupon its failure causes the abrupt fall in estrogen and progesterone levels cited above. This results in a withdrawal of the hormonal support of the endometrium, thereby precipitating menstruation. Should pregnancy occur, the corpus luteum's survival is prolonged, estrogen and progesterone levels continue to rise, and menstruation is deferred (see chapter 2).

The BBT chart, therefore, (1) indicates that the hormonal events associated with ovulation have occurred and that the woman presumably released an egg from her ovary and (2) provides a rough idea about when ovulation occurred and the length of the second half of the cycle. Nothing more should be read into the chart, however. It is a misconception that the BBT chart can precisely pinpoint the ideal time for intercourse.

The cervical mucus begins to thicken rapidly a few hours following ovulation and becomes almost impenetrable to sperm within 24 to 48 hours after ovulation. As the temperature rises around the same time, the likelihood that pregnancy will occur when natural intercourse is timed with the temperature rise is remote. Therefore, thinking behind the old scenario of the woman saying "Hurry home, honey, my temperature has risen and we should try and have a baby!" is without foundation. By that time, it will already be too late to get pregnant. It

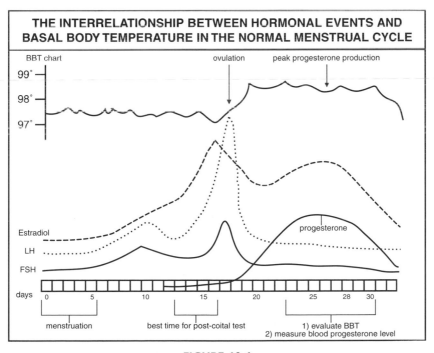

FIGURE 10-1

is far better to time intercourse with the onset of the LH surge as determined by urine testing as the detection of LH in the urine precedes ovulation by eight to 36 hours, a time when the condition of the cervical mucus should be optimal.

Regular menstrual periods.   Regular menstrual periods associated with breast tenderness and, often, mood changes preceding the onset of the periods, and some discomfort (cramping) during menstruation are all clinical indications that the woman is likely to be ovulating.

Urine tests.   Since the surge of the hormone LH triggers ovulation, detection of LH in the urine suggests that ovulation has probably occurred. The woman can easily take this urine test at home around the time of ovulation by performing one of the commercially available home ovulation tests on a sample of her urine. The actual time of ovulation can be predicted by daily, twice daily, or even more frequent performance of the test and charting of the results. It should be kept in mind that there is a two- to four-hour lag before the urine test will reflect the surge of LH in the bloodstream (see figure 10-1).

LH blood-hormone test.   An LH blood-hormone test done several times daily around the time of presumed ovulation (at least 14 days prior to the menstrual period, or when the temperature goes up) is a relatively sophisticated indicator of likely ovulation. This is related to the fact that the LH surge in the middle of the cycle precedes ovulation.

When women used to undergo IVF in natural, unstimulated cycles or when they were given clomiphene citrate without hCG (which acts like an artificial surge of LH), it was necessary to measure LH by repeated blood tests. This series of tests was necessary in order to pinpoint the time of expected ovulation so the eggs could be retrieved before they were ovulated into the fallopian tube or abdominal cavity. Today, the dipstick urine tests that measure the excretion of LH are accurate enough. Serial LH blood testing, which is expensive, time-consuming, and painful, has been virtually supplanted by serial urine LH testing to pinpoint ovulation.

Endometrial biopsy.   An endometrial biopsy, which can be performed in a doctor's office, evaluates the condition of the lining of the uterus. In this relatively painless procedure the physician inserts a small curette or suction apparatus into the uterus a few days prior to expected menstruation and removes a sliver of the endometrium for examination under the microscope. If the endometrium is secretory, indicating the effect of the progesterone, it is likely that the woman has already ovulated. A pathologist is frequently able to pinpoint almost to the day when ovulation is likely to have occurred by microscopically examining the secretory endometrium.

It is also possible to determine whether the endometrial sample is appropriately developed for the stage of the menstrual cycle at which it was taken, thus providing yet another parameter of whether ovulation is occurring in the proper hormonal environment. It is important to remember that although estrogen is not measured in this test, progesterone can act only on a lining that has been stimulated by estrogen. So if microscopic examination shows that the endometrium development is in sync in the middle of the luteal phase, it can be assumed that estrogen stimulation was adequate as well. By combining the endometrial biopsy with measurement of blood or urine hormone levels, it is possible to further refine the evaluation of ovulation.

Progesterone blood-hormone test. The most common indicator of presumed ovulation is the level of the blood hormone progesterone in the woman's blood, as measured a few days before her anticipated menstrual period. This test usually will indicate whether or not the woman is likely to have ovulated, again because progesterone is typically only present in significant amounts in the bloodstream after ovulation.

Analysis of both the LH and progesterone values measures not only whether these hormones are present but also the appropriateness of their levels in the blood relative to the time of the cycle (see figure 10-1).

The bottom line. It is important to view all these tests in context. For example, (1) the blood progesterone level of a week or so prior to menstruation may suggest that ovulation has occurred, (2) a microscopic examination of an endometrial biopsy done a few days prior to menstruation might show that the endometrium has responded appropriately to progesterone, and (3) the length of the luteal phase (as gauged from the urine dipstick test or temperature rise on the BBT chart to the onset of menstruation) was 13 to 14 days. This would indicate a good luteal phase (proper length, enough progesterone, and a normal uterine lining).

The opposite situation might be, on day 25 of the cycle: (1) an endometrium typical of day 19, (2) a significantly lower-than-normal progesterone level a week before menstruation, and (3) a luteal phase of about nine days. This would suggest possible corpus luteum insufficiency and/or insufficient stimulation of the endometrium. In this case the luteal phase is too short, the endometrial response is inappropriate for the timing of the cycle, or the hormonal environment is inadequate. The presence of any of these parameters will lead to the diagnosis of an abnormal hormonal environment. Administration of fertility drugs such as clomiphene, hMG gonadotropins, and hCG will often regulate the pattern of ovulation so that most women with such problems can have a reasonable chance of conceiving. Therefore, ovulation problems alone do not require IVF as a solution.

Integrity of the Reproductive Tract

Since pregnancy can occur only when the reproductive system does not inhibit the passage of sperm, eggs, and embryos, an abnormality within the tract is likely to interfere with the woman's ability to conceive. Careful analysis of her medical history, including any previous venereal diseases, infections following the use of an IUD, and the results of previous fertility tests may suggest the presence of an abnormality such as damaged fallopian tubes, endometriosis, or fibroid tumors. However, defects in the reproductive system can only be confirmed through tests such as those outlined below.

Hysterosalpingogram (HSG). The hysterosalpingogram tests the patency of the fallopian tubes and the shape of the uterus. During the HSG procedure the physician injects a dye into the uterus via the vagina and cervix. The dye shows up as a shadow on an X-ray. The HSG can identify a blockage in the fallopian tubes and may also point out some obvious abnormalities inside the uterus. These could include fibroid tumors, scarring, and abnormalities of uterine development that might occur spontaneously or as a result of DES exposure during the woman's own prenatal development.

The major shortcoming of the HSG is that its usefulness is limited to assessing the shape of the uterine cavity and the patency of the fallopian tubes. It is not a reliable method for detecting small surface lesions in the uterine cavity (e.g., polyps, scarring, and small uterine fibroids that protrude into the cavity). Nor does the HSG yield any information about the ovaries. In other words, fertility problems in which the inside of the fallopian tubes and uterus may appear perfectly normal but where the fallopian tubes are unable to retrieve the eggs from the ovaries because of surrounding scar tissue or ovarian tumors cannot be diagnosed by an HSG. Also, an HSG cannot diagnose endometriosis, in which case the fallopian tubes are usually open.

Women who undergo an HSG should be aware that the procedure is relatively painful, often causing severe cramping. In addition, there is about a 2 percent risk that the dye could convert a dormant infection into a full-blown pelvic inflammation. Women should also be aware that infection can be introduced if the procedure is not performed using the proper sterile technique. Finally, because non-water-soluble dyes tend to collect in damaged tubes and produce infection and complications, there has been a move away from using such dyes. However, the iodine solution in both water-soluble and non-water-soluble dyes can also cause reactions.

Laparoscopy.   One way to both assess the patency of the fallopian tubes and examine the pelvic cavity is by inserting a laparoscope through a small incision in the abdomen. Similar to the lighted, telescope-like instrument used during IVF- or GIFT-related laparoscopy, it enables the physician to look inside the abdominal cavity and perform surgery at the same time. The physician can directly visualize the patency of the fallopian tubes during laparoscopy by injecting a colored, water-soluble (noniodine) solution into the uterus through the vagina and cervix, and observing the fluid's passage through the fallopian tubes. It is also possible to microscopically examine the ends of the fallopian tubes through the laparoscope. Conditions such as endometriosis and pelvic adhesions can be diagnosed with confidence only by laparoscopy or laparotomy, which often afford the opportunity for the physician to treat the problem surgically at the same time. Laparoscopy is usually performed as an outpatient procedure with the patient under general anesthesia. Laparoscopy has largely replaced the HSG as the most popular method of assessing the anatomical integrity of the reproductive tract.

Diagnostic laparoscopy. The *diagnostic laparoscopy* is a procedure that can be performed under anesthesia in the outpatient or hospital setting with minimal discomfort for the patient. A thin telescopelike instrument is inserted via the vagina and cervix into the uterine cavity, and carbon dioxide gas or a liquid is injected to distend the cavity and allow direct visualization of its structure.

Falloposcopy. In a procedure known as *falloposcopy* or tuboscopy, the physician can direct (by watching through the laparoscope) a thin fiber-optic catheter through a separate puncture site into one or both of the fallopian tubes at the time of laparoscopy and then examine the tubal lining for adhesions or damage. Falloposcopy even enables the expert reproductive physician to perform surgery inside the fallopian tubes through the falloposcope, thus avoiding the need to open the abdominal cavity except for the small puncture site. During the same procedure the physician can examine the ovaries as well as the exterior of the fallopian tubes and uterus to see if endometriosis, inflammation, or any other anatomic defect might be contributing to the woman's infertility. However, this procedure is not widely used.

Hysteroscopy. *Hysteroscopy* is a procedure where a telescopelike instrument is inserted via the vagina through the cervical canal into the uterine cavity for evaluation of the interior of the uterus. It is an important procedure because it allows for diagnosis and treatment of surface lesions inside the uterine cavity that adversely affect the ability of an embryo to attach to the uterine lining. Such lesions are often missed in the performance of an HSG.

Surgical procedures to correct defects can be done hysteroscopically. This usually requires prior distension of the uterus with a fluid. Laser-directed procedures can also be performed through the hysteroscope, thereby reducing the chance of bleeding. Therapeutic hysteroscopy has eliminated much of the need for major abdominal surgery, along with its incumbent risks.

Diagnostic hysteroscopy. *Diagnostic hysteroscopy* is performed in the office under intravenous sedation, general anesthesia, or paracervical block, with minimal discomfort to the patient. This procedure involves the insertion of a thin, lighted, telescopelike instrument known as a hysteroscope through the vagina and cervix into the uterus in order to fully examine the uterine cavity. The uterus is first distended with a sterile clear solution (usually physiologic saline) or with carbon dioxide gas, which is passed through a sleeve adjacent to the hysteroscope.

The diagnostic hysteroscopy facilitates examination of the cervical canal and the inside of the uterus under direct vision for defects that might interfere with implantation. Conditions such as fibroid tumors, polyps, bands of scar tissue, or congenital abnormalities can readily be detected. Because we have observed that approximately one in eight candidates for IVF has lesions that require attention prior to undergoing IVF in order to optimize the chances of a successful outcome, we strongly recommend that all patients undergo hysteroscopy or the performance of an FUS exam (see below) so that any lesions so detected can be treated surgically before initiating ART.

Therapeutic hysteroscopy. *Therapeutic hysteroscopy* requires general anesthesia and should be performed in an outpatient surgical facility or conventional operating room where facilities are available for laparotomy, a procedure in which an incision is made in the abdomen to expose the abdominal contents for diagnosis. Therapeutic hysteroscopy is usually combined with laparoscopy.

Fluid ultrasonography (FUS). *Fluid ultrasonography* (FUS), or *sonohysterogram*, is a simple and relatively painless procedure whereby a sterile solution of saline is injected via a catheter through the cervix and into the uterine cavity. The fluid-distended cavity is examined by vaginal ultrasound for any irregularities that might point to surface lesions such as polyps, fibroid tumors, scarring, or a uterine septum.

FUS is highly effective in identifying even the smallest intrauterine lesions and can supplant diagnostic hysteroscopy in the preparation of women for IVF. Moreover, FUS is much less expensive than, less traumatic than, and equally effective as diagnostic hysteroscopy. The only disadvantage lies in the fact that if a lesion is detected, treatment of the problem may require the subsequent performance of hysteroscopy anyway.

Tuboscopy. Tuboscopy is a recently introduced procedure in which a thin fiber-optic telescope is passed into the fallopian tube(s) to evaluate the inner structure.

Other corrective surgery to correct anatomical defects. In most cases, the physician would first attempt to correct defects in the reproductive tract by the least traumatic form of surgery, probably through the laparoscope or hysteroscope. Today almost all pathologic conditions of the uterus, fallopian tubes, or surrounding structures that compromise fertility are accessible to laparoscopic or hysteroscopic surgical treatment. Except for women under 35 who have had a tubal ligation for sterilization purposes, any anatomical defect that cannot be corrected using the laparoscope or hysteroscope probably requires IVF. Laparotomy for tubal disease is fast becoming a thing of the past.

The advisability of corrective surgery on the fallopian tubes depends on the situation. If a young woman has had a tubal ligation for the purpose of sterilization and now wants her fallopian tubes reconnected, tubal microsurgery may be her best option, depending on whether (1) the entire tube was destroyed in the process, (2) there is enough of the tube remaining on either end to allow reconnection, (3) the fimbriated ends of the fallopian tubes are intact, and (4) previous surgery has caused scarring around the tube that inhibits normal egg pickup by the fimbriae.

Condition of the Cervical Mucus

Cervical mucus insufficiency causes about 5 percent of all infertility problems. Some of the causes of cervical mucus problems include previous surgery for cervical cancer, which sometimes destroys the mucus-producing glands of the cervix, and excessive freezing (cryocautery) of the cervix because of lesions, early cancer, or exposure to drugs such as DES while the woman was inside her mother's womb. Women with DES exposure will likewise also be unable to produce a lush endometrial lining in spite of normal ovulation and normal blood estrogen levels prior to ovulation.

Mucus evaluation at ovulation.   The simplest way to evaluate the cervical mucus is to examine the woman around the time of presumed ovulation. At the appropriate time the physician inserts a speculum in the woman's vagina, retrieves some cervical mucus, and evaluates the physical-chemical properties that normally occur in the mucus at ovulation. Healthy cervical mucus should be clear, stringy (stretchy), and should form a fernlike pattern when dry.

Postcoital test (PCT), or Hühner test.   At the same time the physician may conduct a postcoital test (PCT), or Hühner test, to assess the interaction of the mucus and sperm. The woman should have intercourse from six to 18 hours before her appointment. Then the physician will take a mucus sample from her cervical canal via a catheter and examine the mucus on a slide under the microscope.

The PCT assesses the number of sperm in the mucus and evaluates their motility. The presence of a large number of sperm moving in a linear and purposeful fashion usually indicates that the mucus is healthy. The PCT is a good screening test because it provides a rough evaluation of the quality of the sperm as well as of the cervical mucus. At the same time, a less favorable postcoital test does not necessarily indicate a cervical-mucus deficiency because the sperm could be at fault. It should be borne in mind that the most common causes of a poor postcoital test are the following:

1.   Poor timing of the test. If the test is performed more than 12 hours after ovulation has occurred, the cervical mucus may have become thick and tenacious, thereby preventing the invasion of sperm. Accordingly, the postcoital test should be performed immediately prior to or at the time of ovulation. The best method of ensuring that the timing is correct is by performing daily home ovulation urine testing,

which will show a color change eight to 36 hours prior to the occurrence of ovulation

2. Male infertility because the male partner has a low sperm count

3. Inflammation of the cervix (cervicitis) due to ureaplasma, chlamydia, or other organisms

4. The presence of sperm antibodies in the woman's or the man's reproductive secretions

5. Destruction or absence of the cervical glands because of surgery or infection, which will limit the amount of cervical mucus produced and also adversely affect its quality, thereby yielding a poor postcoital test

6. The prior use of clomiphene citrate for more than three consecutive months. In the case of clomiphene citrate being used in women over 40, a hostile cervical mucus is often observed in the very first cycle of stimulation

7. A DES abnormality of the reproductive tract (see chapter 9), which is commonly associated with poor mucus production

Tests of the cervical mucus and blood for antibodies. If analysis of the cervical mucus at ovulation and a postcoital test are not sufficient, the physician may look for sperm antibodies in the cervical mucus and blood. In such cases it may be necessary to culture the mucus or analyze the blood for various microorganisms that might have destroyed the cervical glands' ability to produce the proper mucus.

THE BASIC INFERTILITY WORKUP

Tests Performed on the Woman at Specific Times in the Cycle

1. On the third day of a spontaneous or progesterone-withdrawal menstruation, blood is drawn for the measurement of estradiol, FSH, LH, and inhibin-B.

2. Blood should also be drawn (anytime) for the measurement of prolactin, TSH, and antisperm antibodies (ASA).

3. Commencing on the second day of the menstrual cycle, a BBT chart should be initiated. A thermometer is placed in the mouth for a period of two minutes upon awakening (prior to the ingestion of food/liquid and toothbrushing), and the temperature should be documented graphically on the BBT chart provided.

4. *For women under 35 years of age without evidence or symptoms suggesting underlying organic pelvic disease (e.g., endometriosis, chronic inflammation, pelvic adhesions, fibroids):* A hysterosalpingogram (HSG) should be performed within a week of the cessation of menstruation. This outpatient procedure involves injection of a radio-opaque dye which outlines the fallopian tubes, allowing the diagnosis of tubal blockage. To a lesser degree, it permits the detection of surface lesions inside the uterine cavity. (See HSG subsection earlier in this chapter.)

OR

For all women over 35 and for younger women who have symptoms or signs suggesting underlying organic pelvic disease (e.g., endometriosis, chronic inflammation, pelvic adhesions, fibroids): A laparoscopy/ hysteroscopy should be performed within a week of the cessation of menstruation.

5. Commencing approximately 16 days before the onset of the next expected menstrual period (i.e., usually about 11 days following the initiation of menstruation), urine should be collected twice daily and tested for the onset of the spontaneous LH surge, which usually precedes ovulation by eight to 36 hours. In order to detect the onset of the LH surge as early as possible, it is important that urine be tested at least twice daily. This is done as follows:

The bladder is emptied first thing in the morning, upon awakening. One half-hour later, urine is collected (only a very small amount is required) and tested using an over-the-counter LH kit. The earliest sign of any color change should be documented. It need not be a pronounced color change as suggested by the insert in the kit; any alteration in color is significant. The same process of testing is then repeated at night before retiring. At the earliest sign of a color change:

- The couple should have intercourse and arrange to undergo the first in-office physician's assessment within six to 18 hours following intercourse.

- The woman should *proceed directly* the physician's office to have her blood drawn for the measurement of estradiol. *Timing is critical* because approximately six hours following the detection of LH in the urine (which roughly coincides with 12 hours after the actual onset of the LH surge), blood estradiol levels often start to fall precipitously; and if blood is drawn too late, the measurement of estradiol will be of little value. *If the color change is observed in the early morning,* the woman should schedule the first in-office assessment at the doctor's office for the afternoon of the same day. *If the color change occurs at night,* the doctor's office should be contacted first thing the next morning, and the first in-office assessment should take place within hours.

The first in-office assessment.

A. **A postcoital test (PCT), or Hühner test** is performed on the cervical mucus. The purpose of the PCT is to assess sperm survival within the mucus. Since sperm can only survive for six hours in the vagina, a positive PCT is indicative of:
    1. Good-quality sperm
    2. Good sperm-cervical mucus interaction, suggesting that there will be safe passage of sperm to the uterine cavity
    3. Absence of ASA antibodies in the sperm or mucus
    4. An adequate production of estrogen
    5. The endometrial lining being well primed by estrogen, which is essential for adequate preparation of the uterine lining for implantation

B. **Cervical mucus is cultured for:**
    1. Ureaplasma urealyticum (this requires a specialized medium to transport the specimen to the laboratory)
    2. Chlamydia and gonococcus (these also require a specialized transport medium)
    3. Aerobic and anaerobic pathogens

C. **Cervical mucus is evaluated:** A sample of the cervical mucus is allowed to dry on a glass slide and is examined under the microscope for specific features such as "ferning," which indicates an adequate estrogen effect.

D. **A vaginal ultrasound examination** is performed to detect the presence of at least one dominant follicle that measures 18 millimeter in mean diameter, thus helping to confirm that ovulation is imminent. It also allows for assessment of the thickness and appearance of the endometrial lining. A normal endometrium should measure at least 9 millimeters in sagital diameter at this time.

The second in-office assessment.   The second in-office assessment is scheduled three days after the first office assessment. On the second visit, a vaginal ultrasound exam is performed to determine whether ovulation has occurred. The presence of a small amount of fluid in the lowest region of the pelvis or a change in the shape of the follicle is suggestive of ovulation.

The third in-office assessment.   At the third in-office assessment, which takes place five days after the second in-office assessment, blood is drawn for the measurement of progesterone and estradiol.

The fourth (and final) in-office assessment.   During this final visit, five days after the third in-office assessment, an endometrial biopsy is performed. (See description of endometrial biopsy earlier in this chapter.)

Intercurrent testing (i.e., any time in the cycle) on the woman.

1.   An immunologic workup may be required in certain cases of female infertility or where there is a past history of recurrent pregnancy loss. It includes measurement of antiphospholipid antibodies (APA), antithyroid antibodies (ATA), reproductive immunophenotype (RIP), and a natural killer cell activity test (NKa).

2.   For women who anticipate going into an IVF cycle sometime in the near future, blood should be drawn for the measurement of HIV, hepatitis B surface antigen, hepatitis C antibody, RPR (a syphilis test),

blood grouping, and RH testing as well as a rubella antibody test. Such tests will usually not be required in the course of a routine basic infertility workup; their performance should be confined to cases where it is anticipated that ART procedures such as IVF or GIFT will be the primary approach.

Tests on the Male Partner

1.   A semen analysis is required for accurate measurement of sperm motility and count. Sperm morphology is assessed employing "Kruger criteria." Semen should also be cultured for ureaplasma urealyticum, chlamydia, gonococcus, and for aerobic/anaerobic pathogens
2.   Sperm DNA integrity assay (SDIA)
3.   Antisperm antibodies (ASA)
4.   If IVF is being considered, the man should also undergo blood testing for hepatitis B surface antigen, hepatitis C antibodies, syphilis, and HIV

IVF SHOULD BE CAREFULLY WEIGHED
AGAINST ALL OTHER OPTIONS

Factors that should be considered when deciding between alternative procedures and IVF include (1) success rates of the various procedures, (2) financial considerations, (3) physical toll, (4) emotional investment, and (5) the insistent ticking of the biological clock, which may mandate quick action if ovarian failure for the woman is imminent.

With alternatives to IVF, especially surgical options, a woman is usually given long-range hope: "Now that you've had your operation, let's see how you do in the next two to three years." There is always the possibility that during those 24 to 36 months she will not conceive. And gradually coming to terms with failure in such circumstances is an easier, slower adjustment than it would be with IVF. With IVF, the time frame is compressed into one month; and when a couple fails to conceive during one treatment cycle, they know immediately they have nothing to show for their efforts. The emotional impact is far greater with IVF. It is abrupt and painfully traumatic. Accordingly, couples should decide whether other alternatives that require a lengthy period of anticipation might be more appropriate for them before embarking on IVF. But when couples choose IVF over other assisted reproductive technologies, the rewards can be great.

The following comments from two first-time parents in their mid-forties describe how repeated failures at pregnancy shaped their attitude toward IVF:

Husband: We started trying to have a baby when there wasn't anything like IVF available. We went through all the different fertility tests, and sometimes we gave up temporarily and then decided to try again. We had a lot of disappointments.

Wife: If it hadn't been for my husband I would never have tried IVF, because I was so tired of being let down. But he said if you don't try you have nothing. It was hard emotionally to go through IVF, to relive those hopes and risk getting hurt again, but I'm so glad I did. We have a three-month-old daughter now who has dramatically changed our lives.

11

SHAPING REALISTIC EXPECTATIONS ABOUT IVF

Procreation—and with it the ability to achieve immortality by living on through one's children—is an inalienable right as well as one of the most insatiable human needs. This strong natural urge exerts tremendous pressure on couples unable to have a baby. And the pressure to reproduce becomes increasingly acute as couples grow older and become more aware of their own mortality.

Although IVF offers hope to many infertile couples who until recently had no way of conceiving, it is not a panacea for every couple who want a baby. In addition, every IVF procedure exacts an emotional, physical, and financial price from both partners. No one gets through the process without paying the toll. All couples considering IVF should learn what they can reasonably expect from it before they commit to the procedure. Once they have shaped realistic expectations about their probable experiences, they are ready to decide whether IVF is truly for them.

WHAT ARE A COUPLE'S REALISTIC CHANCES OF SUCCESS?

The following profile fits the ideal candidate/couple for IVF:

1. The woman is under 39
2. The egg provider has at least one healthy ovary capable of responding normally to fertility agents (a low FSH and a normal Inhibin B on the third day of the cycle)

3.   The uterus and endometrial lining of the embryo recipient are normal and capable of sustaining a healthy pregnancy

4.   The egg provider has been pregnant in the past, thereby proving that her eggs can fertilize

5.   There are no immunologic impediments to implantation

6.   The sperm provider has motile sperm and a normal SDIA

These criteria are not absolute, however. For example, in many cases the adverse effect of advancing age on egg and hence embryo quality could in part be offset by transferring a greater number of embryos to the woman's uterus, thereby permitting natural selection to determine which embryos are healthy enough to implant. Alternatively, the application of advanced technologies such as assisted fertilization through ICSI might promote fertilization in cases associated with sperm dysfunction, or assisted hatching might possibly improve implantation potential in cases where the zona pellucida enveloping the embryo is too thick or resistant, as is now believed to occur with advancing age.

Here is a practical example. Let's say a woman is 34 years old, her partner has normal sperm function, and following stimulation with fertility drugs eight eggs are retrieved from her ovaries. She has a normal uterine cavity, as assessed by FUS, and an excellent endometrial lining, as evaluated by ultrasound. Such a woman would, in an optimal IVF setting, have about a 50 percent chance of having a baby following a single IVF cycle of treatment.

Now, if the same woman had a male partner with sperm dysfunction, but by employing ICSI the physician was able to transfer two good quality embryos to her uterus, she could be expected to have the same chance of getting pregnant regardless of male infertility. High technology, by improving the chances of fertilization, has offset the adverse effect of sperm dysfunction on outcome.

Here is another example. Let's say the woman is 40 years old with (apart from her age) exactly the same optimal circumstances as the younger woman described above. Her chances of pregnancy would be significantly reduced because of the adverse effect of age on egg and embryo quality. Her chances of having an IVF baby after one attempt in the same setting would be about 30 percent if three good-quality cleaved embryos were transferred. Here, an age-related embryo-quality deficiency has been partly offset by transferring a greater number of embryos. It could be argued that she might have a strong chance of a multiple pregnancy if so many embryos were put into her uterus. But this is not necessarily the case because most of her embryos would likely be compromised by age and thus would be rejected by her uterus through the natural selection process. Effectively, only three out of the eight embryos might be healthy enough to produce a baby. (See chapter 8 for a discussion of the effect of age on multiple-pregnancy rates.)

Therefore, couples who are contemplating IVF should initially base their realistic expectations for success on those criteria that have the potential to predict outcome, and then temper their expectations with the realization that many of the adverse factors can be partially overcome. However, it is not always possible to overcome severe deficiencies. For example, embryos may never be able to implant into a uterus with surface lesions, such as fibroid polyps that protrude into the uterine cavity, or severe scarring in the uterine cavity due to previous infection. Such conditions would interfere with implantation.

Each couple and their physician, then, must assess these criteria, given their own unique set of circumstances and the environment of the IVF program they have selected, to determine their own realistic expectations of getting pregnant.

THE COUPLE MUST BE SURE THEY ARE TRYING TO CONCEIVE FOR THE RIGHT REASONS

Both partners owe it to themselves, each other, and their unborn child to examine what they expect to achieve from parenthood and what they are willing to contribute before they get on the IVF roller coaster. Successful parenting is usually rooted in a stable relationship and a sincere desire for children. An infertile couple who embark on IVF without first considering their motivation can end up with problems even worse than the infertility problem that brought them into IVF in the first place. The addition of a baby to a troubled relationship will compound existing problems as well as create new ones.

Some childless women/couples get caught up in the pursuit of pregnancy because they have an idealized picture of what it would be like to have a baby. They are so intent on proving they can conceive that they lose sight of how their lives will change when a baby becomes part of the family. They may not fully consider whether they are willing to adapt their lifestyle to accommodate a child's demands on their time, energy, mobility, and financial situation—from babyhood on. They must be sure they are not trying to have a child to please someone else—a mother who has always wanted a grandchild, for example. Each partner should feel comfortable knowing that it is okay not to have children at all if either or both prefer to be child-free. Granted, it is often difficult to come to terms with family and societal pressures, but it can be done.

But when a woman/couple want(s) a baby for the right reasons, family and friends are likely to share in the joy over the baby's birth. As one new IVF mother reported:

We've had nothing but total support from our entire family. They call Caryn the "miracle baby." Friends I went to high school with have called or sent cards, and people I don't even know have sent gifts. We're very proud that we went through IVF and that she's here.

The woman's mother expressed her feelings about her daughter's IVF experience with these words:

My daughter tried for seven years to get pregnant. I was beginning to feel I was never going to have a grandchild, and I worried through the whole nine months of her pregnancy. But IVF was marvelous for all of us. It was very exciting, very satisfying.

The woman's father, who was concerned about the procedure's effect on his daughter, was won over after the baby's birth:

My daughter had undergone tubal reconstruction and laparoscopies and so much pain that I thought if IVF failed it would be so defeating for her. I wondered if it was going to be worth it. Of course now I can see that it was well worth it. I just didn't want to see her undergo any more traumas.

And the new mother's best friend told us:

When you have friends who have had infertility problems for years, you suffer with them. You feel guilty about the pleasure you're having from your own family every time they come to visit. So we all feel like Caryn is our baby. She's theirs, but they still have to share her because we've shared all the pain with them.

Couples who choose IVF for the right reasons are likely to reap the greatest rewards from parenthood. They are often the most committed of all parents because they are making the greatest sacrifice to have a baby.

IVF IS AN EMOTIONAL, PHYSICAL, AND FINANCIAL ROLLER-COASTER RIDE

The biggest decision an infertile couple will ever make in regard to IVF is whether or not they really want to become parents. Once they agree that they are committed to parenthood, they must next decide whether they are ready to deal with the emotional, physical, and financial consequences of their actions.

Both Partners Must Share in the Emotional Cost

An IVF procedure requires an enormous emotional commitment at each level of the program, whether or not IVF is successful. This has a permanent impact on the couple. Because the toll can be so great, both partners must be committed to supporting each other from the very beginning.

Based on the statistics reported by our program at the time of this writing, approximately 45 to 50 percent of women under the age of 39 (mean age of 36 years) who undergo IVF at our program will likely have a baby following a first attempt at embryo transfer. For women between 39 and 43, the comparable success rate is about 20 to 30 percent. The success rate falls so sharply after age 43 (to single digits) that these women would probably be best advised not to undergo IVF with their own eggs and to resort to ovum donation instead.

The comparable chance of a baby being born following one cycle of IVF performed in an optimal setting using donor eggs (provided the donor is younger than 35 and the recipient has a normal uterine cavity) is about 50 to 55 percent, regardless of the birth mother's age. The success rate for the second attempt is about the same as for the first. Success rates tend to decline after the third failed attempt.

Only a decade ago the existence of sperm dysfunction roughly halved the anticipated success rates in all age categories and circumstances. However, since the introduction of ICSI, good IVF programs are achieving the same success with IVF performed in cases associated with even the most severe degree of sperm dysfunction as when the procedure is undertaken using normal sperm. ICSI has virtually leveled the playing field. Some women who fail on the first three tries do in fact get pregnant after four or more attempts. Therefore, it is realistic to be optimistic—guardedly, cautiously optimistic. But the couple should also be realistic enough to prepare themselves emotionally so that they are not overwhelmed by failure in case IVF does not succeed.

The IVF Procedure Is Stressful

Both partners should be prepared to respond to a variety of emotionally stressful demands as they undergo IVF:

1.   Dealing with the general stress "baggage" (shame, guilt, anxiety, depression, anger) they bring into the program because of their long-standing battle with infertility

2.   Following new procedures; interacting with a strange and sometimes impersonal clinical staff, perhaps with a constantly changing cast of characters

3.   Living in an unfamiliar environment: different state or country (many couples travel from another state or country to undergo IVF in

a good program), different daily schedule, time-zone changes, separation from their normal support network

4.   Coping with the unpredictable emotions that the fertility drugs trigger in the woman

5.   Reacting to family and marital stress, which may be heightened by the constant need for mutual support

6.   Managing the financial aspects of the procedure

Couples react to the demands of IVF in strikingly different ways. One expectant mother thought the stimulation phase of her second IVF treatment cycle (her first cycle had ended in an ectopic pregnancy) was the most stressful:

One of the most difficult things I went through was the roller-coaster ride waiting for the estradiol level. Would it be high enough? Would I have enough eggs? Would I have to be on another day of fertility injections? It was really the most exhausting part of the entire process.

Fortunately, she produced three eggs and had two embryos transferred (as opposed to five during the first attempt), and she was six months pregnant at the time of this interview.

The mother of a one-month-old IVF son also found the waiting to be most trying:

The expectation between each step was difficult for me. But waiting for the pregnancy test—that was the hardest part!

In contrast, the mother of IVF triplets said:

I was at the point of giving up, and then found new hope through IVF. I was so excited—exhilarated—through the whole process that the time just flew by.

IVF-related stress cannot be entirely avoided, but it can be mitigated by a staff that helps normalize or demystify the experience as much as possible. The creation of an environment where all the couples are "like me" can be encouraging to the anxious IVF couple. In addition, the opportunity to talk with other couples undergoing the procedure or with representatives of a support group may be helpful. Finally, the services of an in-house counselor can be particularly beneficial.

A Realistic Attitude toward Miscarriage

It is important to remember that the miscarriage rate after IVF is probably no higher than in nature. The reason the IVF miscarriage rate sometimes appears to be higher is that an IVF pregnancy is diagnosed long before it normally would be in the case of a natural pregnancy. Most women who conceive on their own do not test themselves for pregnancy until they have missed their period, whereas with IVF the diagnosis of pregnancy is made before the woman misses a period. One should remember, however, that a pregnancy is not confirmed until the presence of a gestational sac has been diagnosed by ultrasound. If this criterion is used to verify pregnancy, then the miscarriage rate with IVF is no greater than that of the population at large.

Painful as it is to the couple, miscarriage can have a positive side. It is reasonable to expect that although a successful pregnancy was not possible on the first try, the fact that they proved they could initiate a pregnancy means that their overall chances of having a baby will increase on subsequent IVF attempts.

A Realistic Attitude toward Ectopic Pregnancy

When an ectopic pregnancy occurs following infertility treatment, the physician should be on the lookout for the earliest possible signs of trouble (see Chapter 9). The performance of a vaginal ultrasound within two weeks of a positive blood pregnancy (hCG) test following IVF allows for early detection of the unruptured pregnancy and timely intervention with MTX (methotrexate) and/or laparoscopy.

Ectopic pregnancies sometimes occur after IVF when the fluid in which the embryos are ejected from the catheter during embryo transfer drains into a fallopian tube, carrying the embryos with it. The risk of ectopic pregnancy following IVF is only about 3 percent.

Recent advances in the field of ultrasound diagnosis along with the introduction of methotrexate therapy have revolutionized the treatment of ectopic pregnancy and have significantly reduced both the high morbidity and mortality rates previously associated with this condition.

A Realistic Attitude toward Success

Couples must realize that no matter how hard they try to become pregnant, they cannot control the outcome of IVF. There is nothing they can do to influence whether they succeed or fail. When couples become so intent on trying to conceive that they lose sight of the other aspects of their relationship, one clinical coordinator reminds her patients to "lighten up" a bit by writing them prescriptions for candlelight and wine.

The father of triplets, meeting with a group of other IVF couples, commented:

All of us have one thing in common—we've been through the highs and lows of IVF. My wife and I represent the high! But it wasn't always easy for us. I can't emphasize enough how important it is for everyone to keep their chin up through the whole procedure.

Another man, holding his one-month-old son in his arms, added:

I would encourage everyone definitely to maintain a positive attitude. The hardest part of the whole procedure is dealing with failures. It's inevitable that when the first IVF attempt fails you just stop wanting to try because you don't want to fail again. If you could just keep it in perspective and know IVF is a trial-and-error scientific procedure and sometimes you just have to expect problems, that will help a great deal.

A Realistic Attitude toward Failure

It is important for couples to realize that there is little the woman can do to influence outcome following IVF in either a positive or negative way. Women often tend to blame themselves when they get a negative result. This is almost always unfounded and counterproductive, but it is also unfortunately relatively inevitable. Appropriate counseling and a good emotional support system can go a long way toward minimizing this misperception.

Coping with IVF's Physical Demands

The physical demands of IVF range from the annoyance of hormone shots and blood tests to the discomfort of egg retrieval for the woman and the need for the man to produce a semen specimen on demand. The couple probably will have undergone a variety of diagnostic procedures to determine the reason for their infertility and thus may already be familiar with some of these demands.

Certainly when compared with tubal surgery, the process of ultrasound egg retrieval presents a minimal degree of risk, discomfort, and complications. However, it is still an emotionally and physically draining experience. In addition, if the woman has selected a program in another state or country, she may undergo additional physical discomfort as a result of the stress of travel, including jet lag and the general disorientation caused by temporarily living in unfamiliar surroundings.

Proper emotional preparation and mutual support throughout the treatment cycle will help both partners cope more effectively with the physical demands on the woman. And they should keep in mind that once the pregnancy is confirmed, the remainder of the gestational period will probably vary little from pregnancies experienced by all other expectant women.

IVF Requires a Significant Financial Commitment

Until IVF is universally funded by medical insurance in the United States, it will continue to be a program for the haves, not the have-nots. This is true even though its cost only really becomes significant when the woman is wheeled into the operating room for egg retrieval. That is when the fees for anesthesiology, surgery, processing and fertilizing the eggs and sperm, and transferring the embryos mount into thousands of dollars within a few days. Until the egg retrieval, the couple only has to pay relatively minimal costs.

However, the cost of attempting to conceive is not usually limited to the IVF procedure. Many couples have learned how high the overall expenses of attempting to conceive can be. As one newly expectant IVF patient said:

So far we've spent about $80,000 trying to get pregnant, so the IVF portion was really a minor part of the total cost. I first went through reconstructive surgery, then five or six laparoscopies. I shudder to think of the money we spent on airfare to consult with doctors in other cities, plus hotel rooms and meals, to say nothing of all the income we lost by taking so much time away from work. Had we known that my tubes were permanently blocked, we could have saved a lot of money by going directly [to] IVF. But out of that $80,000 our insurance company has paid about $35,000, so we have been pretty lucky financially.

Although this woman considered herself lucky to have paid "only" $45,000 out of her own pocket, a similar outlay would be prohibitive for most other couples. That is why couples contemplating IVF should first determine whether their budget can accommodate all the direct and indirect expenses that IVF entails.

A Realistic Attitude toward Budgeting for IVF

When inquiring about costs at a particular IVF program, the couple should always ask for written quotations that cover all the charges they will incur. This is to avoid any distressing surprises that might be caused, for example, if the program omitted a hefty charge for multiple tests from its price quotation. The couple should not be afraid to ask about items they do not understand.

In addition to the total fee quoted by the program, the couple who must travel from their locality to a program elsewhere should budget generously for the kinds of expenses mentioned above: air or ground transportation, meals, hotels, other travel expenses, allowances for lost income, even baby-sitters or house-sitters while they are on the road. If they plan to visit several IVF programs before selecting one, they should also allow for the expenses they will incur during each site inspection.

In many cases, the couple will have to pay up front for the entire procedure. IVF programs usually request payment in advance in order to avoid problems collecting from the couples who do not get pregnant. Most programs will advise the couple how to bill the insurance company for the reimbursable components of the procedure but will not bill the company directly.

A Realistic Attitude toward Insurance Coverage

Couples should not automatically assume that their insurance will cover the IVF expenses. Reimbursement practices vary from company to company and from state to state. Currently, insurers in less than one-third of the states in the United States offer varying degrees of coverage for IVF. As we have mentioned throughout this book, the attitude of insurance companies with regard to IVF could improve. As one new mother said vehemently:

We're still waiting for our insurance to pay. It's been over a year since we went through the IVF program, and they just keep making excuses. So far we've only received $670!

The father of triplets expressed his concern about the unfairness of insurance companies that refuse to fund IVF but cover other surgical procedures without question:

Through all of our infertility treatments, including artificial insemination and surgeries, the insurance companies argued and refused to pay. Then our triplets were born seven weeks premature, and the hospital bill for them and my wife was $188,000! The insurance company said that was no problem and they were going to pay the whole thing.

The financial risk in IVF is great, but the return can be priceless. That is why it is so important for each couple to be absolutely sure of their willingness and financial ability to make such an investment before they attempt IVF. Yet more and more couples are willing to make the financial commitment. Why? When asked if he and his wife had difficulty deciding whether to undergo IVF given its cost and uncertain outcome, one new IVF father responded:

Well, when you really want children you set your priorities. We think babies are more important than fancy vacations or a sailboat. We were able to budget for IVF. But we're sorry that insurance doesn't usually cover it because a lot of people just can't spend $12,000 to $25,000 or so to go through these procedures.

In chapter 16 we explain in more detail why most insurance companies still do not reimburse for IVF.

HOW MANY TIMES SHOULD A COUPLE ATTEMPT IVF?

Because of the emotional, physical, and financial toll exacted by IVF, it is preferable that no one undertake a one-shot attempt. If a couple can only afford one treatment cycle, IVF is probably not the right procedure for them. After all, in good programs there is still only about a two-in-five chance that IVF will be successful—and there's a tremendous letdown if it fails.

We believe it is unreasonable to undergo IVF with the attitude that "if it doesn't work the first time, we're giving up." IVF is a gamble even in the best of circumstances. But statistically speaking, the ideal IVF candidates who have selected a good IVF program are likely to have a better than 75 percent chance if they undergo IVF three times using their own eggs and an 85 percent chance with donor eggs, as long as their gametes can fertilize, the egg provider is under 39, and the embryo recipient has a normal uterine cavity and a proper hormonal environment.

Unfortunately, some people are destined to remain childless. In our opinion, it is rarely advisable to undergo IVF more than four times in a reputable IVF program that gets good results. After that, the time may have come to consider other options, such as ovum donation, IVF surrogacy, or adoption. However, there are indeed exceptions. One of the authors (GS) recently had a case where a woman of 42 years who had undergone 22 failed attempts at IVF elsewhere had a baby (using her own eggs) on her first attempt with us. This was likely due to the ultimate detection of a treatable immunological problem. In our opinion, therefore, the time to stop doing IVF would not simply be based upon the number of prior failed attempts. Rather, it should hinge upon whether a potentially treatable reason for the prior IVF failures can be identified.

One woman, who eventually adopted a newborn boy, described her disappointment over three failed procedures:

It's very difficult to deal with. You go into any of these procedures with the expectation they will work. Somehow we are raised in our society to think that it's not whether you are going to have children, but how many do you want? We plan for our car, and we plan for our house—and assume that the children are going to come. And when they don't, it's devastating. You are basically out of control of your own body.

Couples who choose to undergo IVF should realize from the outset that the inability to become pregnant should never be considered a reflection on them as individuals. They should view the entire procedure with guarded optimism but nevertheless must be emotionally prepared to deal with the ever-present possibility of failure.

COUPLES MUST CONSIDER THE POSSIBILITY OF A MULTIPLE PREGNANCY

As we mentioned earlier, the couple who are unwilling to settle for a low pregnancy rate must be prepared for the possibility of multiple offspring. With IVF, twins are born in 35 percent of pregnancies and triplets in 5 percent. Compare this to twins once every 80 births and triplets once every 6,000 in natural spontaneous conceptions. It is important to distinguish between the number of multiple births (being discussed here) and the number of multiple pregnancies. This is because most women who are carrying more than twins will opt for pregnancy reduction. Also, many multiple pregnancies reduce spontaneously.

Because the incidence of larger, more hazardous multiple pregnancies is higher with IVF, the couple should be familiar with the concept of selective pregnancy reduction. This trade-off between pregnancy rate and the possibility of multiple births is one of the most important issue involving realistic expectations that couples must resolve.

Selective Reduction of Pregnancy

Some women, because of uterine pathology (e.g., multiple fibroids), surgery, congenital abnormalities, or prenatal exposure to DES, are at risk of premature labor even with a singleton pregnancy. For many such women, carrying twins would likely present an unacceptable risk. However, most women undergoing IVF can usually tolerate and many even covet a twin pregnancy.

A high-order multiple pregnancy (triplets or greater) is another matter altogether, since the increased incidence of prematurity poses an inordinate threat to the well-being of the mother and her babies. What is more, the higher the multiple, the greater the hazard. For the mother, risks include: high blood pressure, uterine bleeding, and surgical complications associated with a cesarean section. For the babies, the risks relate primarily to premature birth; and the higher the multiple, the more premature the birth is likely to be.

It has been determined that in about 40 percent of high-order multiple pregnancies, at least one of the babies is likely to expire or suffer permanently from physical and/or neurologic complications associated with premature birth. For this reason, most IVF programs limit the number of embryos/blastocysts transferred to two or three. In cases where a high-order multiple pregnancy occurs, many programs counsel the couple with regard to selectively reducing the multiple pregnancy down to twins and in certain cases, to a singleton. In such circumstances, selective pregnancy reduction could be regarded as a morally justifiable decision aimed at optimizing the quality of life after birth. Furthermore, given the heart-rending nature of the decision, selective pregnancy reduction might even be considered to be laudable.

Selective reduction of pregnancy is usually performed prior to completion of the third month of gestation. It involves the injection of a chemical, under guidance by ultrasound, directly into one or more developing concepti so as to reduce the total number (usually to twins). This is soon followed by absorption of the products of conception by the body. Properly performed by an expert, selective reduction of pregnancy, rarely (2–7 percent of cases) results in total loss of the pregnancy.

SOME COUPLES MAY HAVE MORAL/ETHICAL/RELIGIOUS OBJECTIONS TO IVF

While a discussion of the moral, ethical, and religious dilemmas created by IVF is not within the scope of this book, we would encourage all couples to come to terms with their concerns in this regard before entering an IVF program. No one should be excluded from an IVF program because of religion any more than because of age, race, marital status, or sexual preference. Every case should be assessed on its own merit. The couple should be willing to discuss concerns openly with their physician; the IVF program staff; and their minister, priest, rabbi, or mullah. Sometimes, by working together, it is possible to find approaches that will satisfactorily resolve everyone's concerns.

MATCHING REALISTIC EXPECTATIONS WITH THE RIGHT PROGRAM

Once the couple forms their own realistic expectations about IVF and have decided to undergo the procedure, it is time to select a program. When evaluating potential programs, the couple should expect an IVF provider to meet three basic criteria: (1) provide the highest quality of medical care, (2) ensure that the couple will have the best possible opportunity of conceiving within the guidelines of sound medical practice, and (3) deal with the couple in a manner consistent with the emotional, physical, and financial investment they will make. The following chapter explains how consumers can evaluate IVF programs on the basis of these characteristics.

12

HOW TO FIND THE RIGHT IVF PROGRAM

The infertile couple (or woman) should begin their search for the right IVF program by talking with their own physician and/or a local fertility support group. If there are no fertility support groups in the area, the couple should contact the national headquarters of one of these organizations. They may also wish to talk to couples who have already undergone IVF, as these couples tend to develop a close network and will probably be happy to share their experiences. Contacts made through such networking will likely lead to even more sources of information.

We wish to stress that no matter how strongly the couple feel that time is closing in on them, it is important to devote a few months to diligent research rather than rushing arbitrarily into the most convenient program.

HOW SHOULD THE SUCCESS OF AN IVF PROGRAM BE EVALUATED?

The process of selecting an IVF program is significantly different from that of choosing a physician, whose credentials alone assure the couple of his or her competence and expertise. First, there is currently no accrediting agency that provides audited outcome-based information to consumers about an IVF program's competence and success.

The couple should evaluate more than the expertise of just one person. They should also take into account the success rate of all the individuals who operate as a team. For example, a laboratory that is not very successful at fertilization would be a drawback in a program that has a friendly, supportive staff and otherwise presents a reliable, innovative image.

How does one gauge the success of an IVF program? In the broadest terms an IVF program's success can be measured by its

1.   **results** (a track record that is consistent with currently accepted rates for successful IVF procedures);

2.   **caring** (the degree to which the couple perceive an attitude of caring manifested by the staff);

3.   **staff interaction** (whether there seems to be open, harmonious interaction among the staff involved in the program, and whether the couple feel comfortable dealing with the staff); and

4.   **reputation** (how the program is regarded by those who have undergone IVF, by the community in which it is situated, by other physicians—and don't forget the program's financial stability).

The only basis for judgment the couple will have when trying to select the most appropriate IVF program is their observation of the way the program operates—from initial contact until patient discharge. In order to properly research individual IVF programs, they will first have to learn to understand and interpret the terms and statistics they will probably encounter.

HOW DOES THE PROGRAM DEFINE PREGNANCY?

The word pregnancy often means different things to different people. For example, the terms *chemical pregnancy* and *clinical pregnancy* are frequently used interchangeably although they have completely different meanings. It's necessary to understand both of these definitions in order to avoid misinterpreting the statistics that may be quoted.

Chemical Pregnancy

Chemical pregnancy refers to biochemical evidence of a *possible* developing pregnancy. A positive blood or urine pregnancy test confirms a chemical pregnancy provided that the woman has not received the hormone hCG recently and does not have a tumor that releases hCG into her blood. (See chapter 7 for a discussion of the quantitative Beta hCG blood pregnancy test.)

Clinical Pregnancy

A clinical pregnancy is one that is *confirmed rather than merely presumed*, as with a chemical pregnancy. A pregnancy can be confirmed when evidence of gestation either in the uterus or fallopian tube is detected by ultrasound and/or when pathological evidence of placental or fetal tissue is obtained following miscarriage or surgery. A blood or urine test alone is not sufficient to confirm a clinical pregnancy.

Chemical vs. Clinical Pregnancy

The couple should keep in mind that only 20 to 30 percent of all naturally conceived pregnancies survive long enough to postpone the menstrual period and thus create the suspicion that the woman is pregnant. This means that most chemical pregnancies never become clinical pregnancies.

Verifying a chemical pregnancy when a woman has undergone IVF is complicated by the fact that she has almost invariably received an injection of hCG at least 11 to 12 days prior to the first Beta HCG blood pregnancy test. Depending upon her body's absorption and excretion rates, small amounts of the hCG may still be present in her blood at the time of the test and could result in the false suggestion of a pregnancy.

Therefore, the term *chemical pregnancy* when applied to IVF rates might mean one of three things: (1) a true chemical pregnancy is present but will not progress to a clinical pregnancy (the most likely scenario), (2) a chemical pregnancy is in the process of developing into a clinical pregnancy, or (3) the result was a false indication of a chemical pregnancy caused by residual hCG.

If the terms *chemical pregnancy* and *clinical pregnancy* are used interchangeably, a quoted pregnancy rate could be falsely inflated, perhaps by as much as 100 percent, by citing the percentage of chemical pregnancies for that particular program. For this reason most reputable IVF programs will not report chemical pregnancies in their statistics.

Consumers should be aware that some programs report "inclusive pregnancy rates," which are clinical and chemical pregnancy rates combined. However, since it is not always possible to determine which terms are actually being quoted when this reporting method is used, couples should not be afraid to ask the proper questions to clarify and distinguish between these two terms.

HOW SHOULD A REPORTED PREGNANCY RATE BE INTERPRETED?

Careful study of and reference to the following two sections on success rates should enable the couple to ask the hard questions of the programs under consideration.

Clinical Pregnancy Rate per Embryo-Transfer Procedure

This refers to the clinical pregnancy rate per embryo transfer performed. Quoting the pregnancy rate on the basis of embryo transfer will inflate the overall results because if no eggs are retrieved or if eggs are retrieved but do not fertilize in the laboratory, the woman accordingly does not undergo an embryo transfer. Thus her case, which actually represents a failed IVF procedure, will not be reflected in the statistics. Had her case been included in the computations, the overall rate would be somewhat lower.

Clinical Pregnancy Rate per Number of Women in the Program

Some IVF programs base their pregnancy statistics on the number of women who undergo the IVF procedure. But to report the pregnancy rate in this manner will inflate results because this method fails to allow for women who may undergo more than one IVF procedure. If the number of patients rather than the number of egg-retrieval procedures performed is used as the statistical base, the success rate will naturally look better.

Clinical Pregnancy Rate per Attempted Egg Retrieval

The variation in statistics that these three definitions can produce is startling. Take a program that is experiencing a 20 percent rate of clinical pregnancies based on the number of egg retrievals performed. If the program instead reports clinical pregnancies on the basis of embryo transfers, its reported results could be 25 percent. Now, if it bases its statistics on the number of clinical pregnancies per number of women patients, it might (depending on the number of times each patient has undergone IVF) quote a success rate of as high as 30 percent. No wonder it is so important to be able to interpret these statistics intelligently. Imagine how these rates could be manipulated even further if the program were to include chemical pregnancies in its computations.

The term *cumulative pregnancy rate* is often used to describe the overall chance of a clinical pregnancy occurring per egg retrieval or per embryo transfer following several successive procedures. Cumulative birthrate refers to the overall chance of a woman having one or more babies per egg retrieval or per embryo transfer following several attempts.

WHAT IS AN ACCEPTABLE SUCCESS RATE?

Birthrate per Egg Retrieval Procedure

While proper reporting of a program's pregnancy rate per egg retrieval reflects the competence of a program, the only statistic that really matters in the final analysis is a woman's chance to have one or more healthy babies per IVF procedure.

We believe that an acceptable success rate is one that is at least as high as the average of the rates being reported at that time from all programs that have experienced a clinical birthrate. Because the mean birthrate per egg retrieval in the United States is about 30 percent for women under 39, based on SART statistics, it is fair to say that a program offering a 30 percent or better chance of a baby being born is operating within the realm of current acceptability.

Birthrate per Embryo Transferred

Since many programs currently limit the number of embryos transferred in order to reduce the incidence of multiple pregnancies, it is both reasonable and appropriate to evaluate performance based on the baby rate per embryo transferred rather than the overall birthrate per IVF procedure. For example, if IVF Program A transfers an average of two embryos to women under 35 years of age while Program B transfers five, then the competency of the programs cannot be compared by the overall success rate. Here, the number of babies born per embryo transferred will give a better indication of performance than the overall pregnancy or birthrate. The national birthrate per embryo transferred for women under 39 years using their own eggs is currently about 15 percent in the United States. The birthrate per embryo transferred will not be 15 percent forever because many programs are improving. However, consumers can expect that the average success rate will increase very slowly.

Anticipated (Probable) Birthrate per Embryo-Transfer Procedure

Because it might take a long time for an IVF program to establish a high success rate based on the number of live babies born, it would be reasonable for a relatively new program to report the anticipated birthrate per embryo-transfer procedure performed. This could be defined as the number of clinical pregnancies per embryo transfer that have progressed beyond the 12th week of gestation plus the number of live, healthy births that have occurred per egg retrieval. The acceptability of this statistic is based on the fact that once a pregnancy has proceeded beyond the 12th week it is highly unlikely to miscarry spontaneously.

In order to compute a mean anticipated embryo-transfer procedure for the United States, several factors must be taken into account. First, it should be kept in mind that the mean IVF clinical pregnancy rate per embryo transfer in women under 39 is about 33 percent. Now, if 10 percent of these pregnancies are lost through early clinical miscarriage and another 5 percent are miscarried after the 12th week, the probable birthrate per embryo transfer would be derived by reducing the 33 percent clinical pregnancy rate by about one-seventh (or 14 percent), so a guesstimate of the anticipated birthrate would be about 29 percent per embryo transfer. Therefore, when investigating a new program that can offer no other statistics, consumers should look for a probable birthrate per embryo transfer of about 29 percent.

We strongly recommend that when asking for success rates the researching couple should hold IVF programs accountable by requesting that they provide all statistics in written form. It is also helpful to ask for long-term statistics (two to three years' worth) to account for the turnover in key staff members that frequently occurs in many IVF programs.

COUPLES HAVE THE RIGHT TO EXPECT COMPETENT, CARING TREATMENT

Another barometer of an IVF clinic's success is the way it treats its patients. A reputable IVF program should help each couple establish rational expectations right from the beginning and then follow through with a professional, understanding, organized program that meets the needs of both partners.

Consumers should look for a program that says, in effect: "We cannot guarantee that you will get pregnant, but we can promise you professionalism, the highest quality of care and expertise, a reasonable chance of getting pregnant, and that you will be treated all along the line with courtesy, understanding, and compassion."

Couples should look for a dedicated, committed team trained to deal with the emotional consequences of an IVF procedure and should avoid a program that is so preoccupied with the technical side of IVF that it loses sight of the human aspects of the procedure. No couple should feel they have to settle for a program that offers poor support and lacks compassion because they have nowhere else to go.

The morale and enthusiasm of the staff are good indicators of the kind of treatment the couple can expect. Morale in clinics that consistently report pregnancies is likely to be higher because staff members feel that they are part of a successful program. One program reinforces this enthusiasm by contacting patients who have a positive pregnancy test via speakerphone. This enables everyone on the staff to share the joy and excitement with the couple.

Consumers might want to look for a program that offers a professional counselor to deal with both partners' emotional needs. The counselor, who is pivotal to any IVF program, usually acts as a buffer between the couple and the clinical team. Counseling can help a couple become positively involved in an IVF program and also steer them away from false hopes.

It is wise to inquire about the size of the staff and verify that the program has enough people to respond to the couple's needs at all times. No one wants to have to reschedule egg retrieval because the doctor in an understaffed clinic was called away unexpectedly.

Care and caring go together in the truly successful IVF program. If the perception of caring truly indicates a successful program, then the program that elicited the following comment from this woman (who adopted a baby after her IVF pregnancy ended in miscarriage) must indeed be successful:

I don't think I'd try IVF again in the very near future because I have a six-week-old at home, but thanks to the staff at the clinic I have a positive attitude and outlook about IVF, and would seriously consider trying again later.

WHAT IS THE BEST WAY TO GET INFORMATION?

The most rational approach to assessing the IVF situation is by first becoming aware of the facts and statistics, asking pertinent questions according to one's own needs, and then actually visiting the site. A reputable program should be willing to answer questions and give the couple access to the facility.

When seeking information about a program, the couple should look for staff who are willing to take the time to talk and to respond to questions frankly and openly. Some consumer-oriented staffs will even send literature about the program on request, as well as copies of articles from accredited professional journals, videotapes, stories about the program from newspapers and magazines, and sometimes names of previous patients who are willing to discuss their experiences.

If the clinic does not volunteer information, the couple may have to be assertive. At a minimum, they should expect to receive literature about how the program operates. The lack of such information for potential patients is a sign of poor organization. The couple should be wary of any program that refuses to provide information and statistics in writing or insists they come into the office. If the couple feel that they have to pry answers from an evasive staff, they should think twice about that program.

Preliminary Information Can Be Obtained by Telephone

The only way to ferret out success rates is by talking directly to someone at the clinic. We recommend that before calling a prospective program the couple should reread "How Does the Program Define Pregnancy?" and "How Should a Reported Pregnancy Rate Be Interpreted?" in this chapter. Then they should be prepared to ask the following questions:

1. How long has your program been established?
2. How many patients have you treated?
3. How many babies have been born?
4. How many egg retrievals have you performed?
5. How many embryo transfers have you done?
6. How many embryos do you transfer at a time?

7. How many clinical pregnancies per egg-retrieval procedure have you recorded?

8. What is your miscarriage rate?

9. (*For established programs*) How many deliveries per embryo-transfer procedure have you reported (birthrate per egg-retrieval procedure)?

10. (*For new programs*) How many deliveries plus ongoing pregnancies that have proceeded beyond the 12th week have you experienced per embryo transfer (anticipated/probable) birthrate per embryo-transfer procedure)?

11. Do you have an embryo cryopreservation program? If so, how successful has it been? (Apply questions 1 through 10 to this issue.)

12. Do you offer ovum donation and IVF surrogacy (when applicable) in your program? (Apply questions 1 through 9 to this query as well.)

13. Do you turn away women over a certain age? If so, what age? (This is to be asked if age is a concern for the couple.)

14. Does your program perform intracytoplasmic sperm injection (ICSI) for the treatment of severe male infertility? How many procedures have been performed, and how many ongoing pregnancies and/or births have occurred?

15. Do you arbitrarily cancel an IVF cycle if there are a "few" mature follicles, or do you include the couple in this decision-making process?

It is the anticipated birthrate statistic that we consider to be the fairest and most helpful because it makes the most recent results available and allows the newer clinics to provide an idea of the probability of having a live birth after IVF is done in their setting. Some consumers might give the benefit of the doubt, at least at first, to new clinics. However, if a program has not been in existence long enough to achieve any pregnancies, the staff should be forthright enough to explain that this is why they have no other statistics to offer.

In order to form the most rational expectations about each program, the couple should attempt to learn how the prognostic indicators for IVF (see chapters 3 and 8) might impact on their personal chance of pregnancy in each particular program. One way to do this would be to direct the conversation to their personal situation after having obtained general statistics about the program. The couple might first offer some information about themselves, including their ages, how long they have been infertile, what has been diagnosed as the cause of their infertility, the status of the man's fertility, and previous surgeries the woman may have undergone to correct her infertility. They should also be willing to supply other information the staff may request in order to become more familiar with the case.

Then the couple might ask:

1. In your program, what would be our chances per embryo transfer of conceiving a clinical pregnancy?

2. What would you say are our chances of actually having a baby after undergoing a single embryo-transfer procedure?

Once again, couples should request the answers to the questions in writing. Thereupon, after narrowing down the list of prospective clinics to those that responded most satisfactorily to these questions, the couple are ready for the next step—the preenrollment interview.

A Preenrollment Interview Is Worth the Time and Expense

Just as few people would select a college without first visiting its campus, consumers also should visit each prospective program if at all possible. A program that refuses to grant a preenrollment interview should be dropped from further consideration.

A preenrollment interview will give the couple a chance to meet some of the staff and see what kind of people they will be dealing with. Is there an air of camaraderie, or do the staff seem disgruntled and unhappy? If the staff obviously regard their positions as nine-to-five drudgery, the couple most likely are in the wrong place.

Is the office comfortable and attractive? Does it create a relaxed, pleasant atmosphere? Does the program provide audiovisual equipment on which patients can watch informational tapes about IVF procedures? Of course audiovisual equipment is not required in order for a woman to get pregnant, but its availability indicates that the clinic cares enough to keep both partners informed and comfortable. A program that offers such amenities is one that cares for the emotional as well as physical needs of its patients.

The couple should try to meet the clinic coordinator during their visit because he or she is the person they will deal with daily. They should be sure the coordinator is in control of the program on a daily basis and will be congenial to work with.

If it is not possible to meet the doctor during the preenrollment interview, the couple might investigate how the doctor is viewed outside the clinic. Does he or she get along well with people? IVF is a popular topic for discussion these days, and many people have strong opinions about the doctors who practice this specialty. The couple may be surprised at how easy it is to get that information.

If a preenrollment interview cannot be arranged, other approaches can be used to gather more information about a specific program. Phone calls to previous patients will be invaluable. The chapter of an infertility support group in the city where the program is located probably would be willing to help. The couple might even retain someone living near the clinic to conduct research for them. Perhaps the couple's own doctor knows a local physician who can provide information. The couple may even decide to randomly telephone some OB-GYNs who practice in that community and ask them about the program.

While such research about a program can be helpful, in most cases nothing can really replace the information gained during a site inspection. A preenrollment trip is well worth the time and expense.

Consumers should expect to do a lot of homework when searching for an IVF program. Unfortunately, we do not believe that it will get any easier in the near future. As an IVF father told us:

We have a library at home of all kinds of clippings, and virtually every book, magazine, and periodical you can imagine about IVF. My wife did a tremendous amount of research on which clinics were having the great-

est success rate, what kinds of procedures were being used, what the latest technology was. Her training as a nurse certainly gave her a better handle on those strange-sounding hormones that are used as part of the process. Really, it was a matter of doing a lot of research for us before we were able to locate the right IVF program.

Helpful as it would be when selecting an IVF program, it is not necessary for every couple to have an RN in the family to use the guidelines suggested in this chapter. When consumers know what to look for and what questions to ask, they will be prepared to make an informed choice—a decision that should always be based on rational expectations, not false hopes.

What about the SART Report?

At the time of writing this book, IVF outcome statistics reported annually by the Society for Assisted Reproductive Technology (SART) lack credibility. The reason is that to date, in spite of public demands and congressional decrees spanning a period of more than two and a half decades, SART has failed to institute a verifiable reporting process by IVF programs. Instead, the IVF outcome data reported annually (hitherto on the CDC Web site) on the SART report comprises outcome data that are largely self-generated by member programs with little or no oversight by SART. For this reason, we do not recommend using the SART report as a method for selecting an IVF program.

13

IUI, GIFT, AND OTHER ALTERNATIVES TO IVF

This chapter outlines some of the therapeutic gamete-related technologies available to the infertile couple. The term *therapeutic gamete-related technologies* refers to those procedures that involve enhancement, insemination, or transfer of eggs and/or sperm into the woman's uterus, fallopian tubes, or peritoneal cavity in the hope that in vivo (inside the body) fertilization and the subsequent birth of one or more healthy babies will follow. In contrast, IVF involves fertilization in the laboratory and transfer into the uterus of embryos/blastocysts rather than gametes.

We will recommend when these technologies should be considered in place of IVF and when IVF would be the best alternative.

ARTIFICIAL INSEMINATION

The procedures mentioned in this section are directed mostly but not exclusively to situations in which infertility is due to problems other than female organic pelvic disease and male-factor infertility. Indications for artificial insemination include cervical mucus insufficiency unrelated to sperm antibodies in the woman's secretions, unexplained infertility, and donor-sperm insemination. It is relatively contraindicated in situations of male-factor infertility, female immunologic infertility (due to sperm antibodies), tubal disease, chronic pelvic adhesions, and for women in their 40s where the chance of having a baby would be less than 4 percent per cycle. Couples for whom artificial insemination is indicated might consider the following alternatives before electing to undergo IVF. IVF would be performed if insemination procedures fail to achieve a pregnancy in spite of repeated attempts.

Intrauterine Insemination (IUI)

Intrauterine insemination (IUI), the injection of sperm into the uterus by means of a catheter directed through the cervix, has been practiced for many years. The premise of this procedure is that sperm can reach and fertilize the egg more easily if placed directly into the uterine cavity.

In the early 1960s, physicians were injecting small quantities of raw, untreated semen (sperm plus the seminal plasma) directly into the uterus at the time of expected ovulation. However, when more than 0.2 ml of semen was injected into the uterus, serious and sometimes life-endangering shock-like reactions often occurred. It was subsequently determined that such reactions were related to the presence of prostaglandins within the seminal plasma. This led to the practice of injecting small amounts (less than 0.2 ml) of raw semen into the uterus. However, the pregnancy rates were dismal; and side-effects, such as severe cramping and infection, were rampant. (Women are protected against the reaction during intercourse because the semen pools in the vagina; the sperm are then safely filtered through the cervical mucus, thereby preventing seminal plasma from reaching the uterine cavity.)

As far back as 1982, we began to recognize the potential advantage of washing and centrifuging raw semen so as to separate sperm from the seminal fluid, and thereby remove the prostaglandins that cause most of the problems. We subsequently introduced and, thereupon, became the first to publish on IUI in the prestigious journal *Fertility and Sterility* (April 1994).

Indications for IUI.
Artificial insemination with cryopreserved donor sperm. The recognition of HIV infection as a sexually transmitted disease, coupled

with the fact that the virus is present in semen months before it can, in most cases, be detected in the blood, mandates that all sperm donors have their semen cryopreserved (frozen) and stored for at least six months, whereupon they will be re-tested for HIV infection. Ideally, only upon confirmation of a negative test should the cryopreserved semen specimen be thawed and used for insemination. Since cryopreservation inevitably reduces sperm motility and function, it is not adequate to simply thaw the frozen specimen and then inseminate the raw semen into the vagina. Rather, the semen specimen should be processed for IUI. Provided that the recipient is ovulating normally, there is no need to administer fertility drugs, such as clomiphene citrate.

The emergence of new tests that can accurately detect HIV without the need to wait for the development of antibodies could change the situation and might in the future again permit the use of fresh sperm.

Artificial insemination with partner's sperm.   In cases of sexual dysfunction (impotence, retrograde ejaculation, etc.) or timing issues, the partner's sperm may need to be collected and processed in preparation for IUI.

Cervical mucus hostility.   Sometimes the cervical mucus acts as a barrier to the activation and passage of sperm as it passes through the cervical canal. This may be due to poor physical qualities of the mucus, cervical infection, or the presence of anti-sperm antibodies. In all but the latter case, IUI can readily be performed during natural cycles unless the woman has ovulation dysfunction. However, when infertility results from the presence of antibodies in the cervical mucus, IUI will likely be ineffectual and should be replaced by IVF.

Abnormal ovulation.   In some cases where the woman requires the use of fertility drugs to induce normal ovulation, the concomitant performance of IUI could optimize pregnancy rates.

The fertility drug of choice, clomiphene citrate (Serophene).   A recent study confirmed that normally ovulating women taking clomiphene citrate experience a reduced chance of achieving pregnancy when compared with fertile women who are not taking clomiphene. Furthermore, additional studies have reported very few viable clomiphene-induced pregnancies in women over the age of 40. The reason is clomiphene's anti-estrogen effect on the lining of the uterus and the production of cervical mucus. The only advantage to clomiphene therapy lies in its simplicity of administration, low incidence of side effects, and relatively low cost. It should also be recognized that clomiphene should not be used for more than three consecutive months without taking a full month's break before starting a fourth cycle of treatment. This is because after the third consecutive month of clomiphene therapy there is a progressive decline in fertility, to the point that following six or more back-to-back cycles of treatment the drug exerts a strong contraceptive influence. This results from a buildup of the anti-estrogenic properties of clomiphene. The good news is that upon discontinuation of clomiphene for six weeks, all of these adverse effects disappear.

Letrazole.   Letrazole, a relatively new oral fertility agent (see chapter 5), works similarly to clomiphene but does not exhibit the same local antiestrogenic effects on the uterine lining and the cervical glands. Accordingly, the selective use of Letrazole might prove to be useful in the performance of IUI.

Gonadotropins.   Women with absent or abnormal ovulation who require fertility drugs in preparation for IUI should receive gonadotropins (e.g., Repronex, Gonal F, Follistim, Bravelle). Granted, these agents are relatively expensive, but they have no anti-estrogenic properties; and in the hands of the experienced physician the pregnancy rate is nearly double that which can be achieved with clomiphene. Side effects can be either prevented or readily managed.

IUI success rates.   Success rates with IUI are contingent upon (1) the procedure being performed for the correct indications, (2) whether the woman is ovulating normally on her own, and (3) the age of the woman. By and large, birthrates per cycle of IUI performed for the correct indications are reported to be about 15 percent for women less than 30 years of age, 12 percent for women 30 to 35 years, 7–8 percent for women 35 to 39 years, and less than 2 percent for women over 40.

Contraindications for IUI.

Refractory male infertility.   Contrary to popular belief, the performance of IUI in cases of moderate or severe male infertility hardly improves success rates over regular and well-timed intercourse alone. IVF with intracytoplasmic sperm injection (IVF/ICSI) is the only method to optimize pregnancy rates in association with male refractory infertility.

Tubal disease.   Since pelvic inflammatory disease (PID) inevitably damages the intricate and sophisticated inner lining of the fallopian tubes, no surgery to the outside of the tube(s) will remedy damage done to the inner lining. As such, the pregnancy rate can be expected to be at least 10 times lower than average when fertility drugs and/or IUI are used in such cases. Moreover, the incidence of ectopic pregnancy is about one in six. Bypassing the "damaged plumbing" with IVF is the only rational treatment is such cases.

Woman's age.   Women over 40 do not have the time to waste on IUI since the success rate is less than 4 percent birthrate per month of trying.

Mild to moderate pelvic endometriosis.   While the exact cause of endometriosis remains an enigma, it is now apparent that a toxic environment exists in the pelvis (surrounding the tubes and ovaries) in patients with this condition. As a consequence, ovulation, whether spontaneous or induced by fertility drugs, commits the egg to pass through a toxic pelvic environment in order to reach the sperm waiting in the fallopian tube. This significantly reduces the egg's fertilization potential. Furthermore, once the fertilized egg reaches the uterus, immunologic factors present in about one-third of cases of endometriosis (regardless of its severity) increase the risk of the embryo being rejected before pregnancy can be diagnosed. Such women may experience repeated "mini-miscarriages." In spite of these antifertility influences, many women with mild endometriosis in fact do conceive on their own or following ovarian stimulation with fertility drugs. However, for reasons already referred to, the chances of conception are significantly reduced; and if the women are ovulating normally on their own, the addition of fertility drugs will afford no additional benefit. Simply put, women in their late 20s to mid-30s, who have the time and inclination to wait, can anticipate about a 30 percent chance of conceiving on their own within three years, contingent upon their ovulating normally and having fertile male partners. The occurrence of pregnancy in the latter cases occurs in spite of, rather than

due to, such treatment. Such women should consider deferring all invasive treatments in favor of a "wait-and-see" attitude. Conversely, for
women over the age of 35 whose egg quality is inevitably on the decline,
IVF offers the only rational approach.

Fertility drugs and multiple births with IUI.   Women who ovulate
normally do not experience much of an increase in multiple birthrates
following ovulation induction, while those with absent or abnormal
ovulation have a higher success rate as well as a much greater multiple
pregnancy rate, often triplets or greater. In an attempt to explain this
observation, we compared and reported on differences in ovarian
response to gonadotropin stimulation between women who ovulate
normally vs. those who have dysfunctional ovulation or do not ovulate
at all. Serial ultrasound examinations around the time of induced ovulation were performed on women undergoing ovarian stimulation with
gonadotropins in preparation for IUI. We observed that normally
ovulating women presented with one and sometimes two follicles significantly larger than the rest (dominant follicles), while the
absent/abnormal ovulators often had numerous large follicles of a similar size. Following the hCG trigger in the normal ovulating group, the
one (and sometimes two) dominant follicle(s) would ovulate while the
remaining follicles did not. Conversely, in absent/abnormal ovulators,
the numerous follicles ovulated. We concluded that in normally ovulating women, once the dominant follicle(s) released the egg(s) the
ovulation of the remaining follicles was blocked.

   Thus, the belief that administration of gonadotropins to normally
ovulating women will trigger the release of multiple eggs and thereby
significantly increase the pregnancy rate is somewhat erroneous.
Neither the multiple pregnancy rate nor the overall pregnancy rate per
cycle is substantially increased in this manner. In contrast, when
gonadotropins are administered to non-ovulating women and/or
women with dysfunctional ovulation, such as women with polycystic
ovarian syndrome (or PCOS, where the ability to select one or more
dominant follicle(s) is absent or compromised, and multiple eggs may
be released), the pregnancy rate per cycle as well as the incidence of
multiple pregnancy is markedly increased.

It follows that only those women with absent or abnormal ovulation are at significant risk of having high-order multiple pregnancies. They, therefore, need to be counseled regarding the consequences of premature birth and the availability of selective pregnancy reduction toward the end of the third month of pregnancy. Another alternative is to avoid the issue completely by choosing IVF, where the number of potential babies can be limited by the number of embryos transferred to the uterus.

It is indeed unfortunate that fertility treatment has become so regimented that most patients find themselves being ushered through a "scripted treatment process," one that almost mandates surgery if the fallopian tubes are damaged or blocked, and clomiphene/IUI for all other cases, even including male infertility. For the majority of couples who require an individualized strategic plan of action at an early stage, such an approach is emotionally, physically, and financially draining, leaving them both suspicious and critical of the intent of the medical profession.

IUI, like any other form of fertility treatment, can be of great value if used appropriately and selectively for the correct indications. The use of fertility drugs should not be regarded as a necessary adjunct in all cases of IUI, which in turn should not be considered as a required preliminary to IVF. Some women are better off with fertility drugs alone, some women require IUI alone, some require IUI with fertility drugs, while others should go directly to IVF.

Intravaginal Insemination (IVI) with Partner's Semen

Intravaginal insemination (IVI) using the partner's semen involves the injection of semen into the vagina in proximity to the cervix rather than into the uterus, as is the case with IUI. Intravaginal insemination is most often employed to assist a woman with a subfertile partner to conceive naturally at the time of ovulation. However, IVI usually offers no advantage over normal ejaculation that occurs during intercourse. The only cases when IVI might be advantageous would be certain forms of male impotence in which the man cannot produce semen with intercourse.

Artificial Insemination by Donor (AID)

Artificial insemination by donor (AID) is the most common form of insemination in cases in which donor sperm is required because the woman's partner is infertile. Artificial insemination by donor can be done via IVI or IUI.

As mentioned under IUI above, the use of cryopreserved donor sperm is the safest method of performing donor insemination, given the significant risk of HIV. After the donor has been tested for HIV, the sperm are cryopreserved for at least six months, following which the donor is retested. If HIV is not present, the likelihood that the original specimen is infected is remote, and the specimen is then released. Again, since cryopreservation inevitably reduces sperm motility and function, it is not adequate to simply thaw the frozen specimen and then inseminate the raw semen into the vagina. Rather, the semen specimen should be processed for AID. Provided that the recipient is ovulating normally, there is no need to administer fertility drugs, such as clomiphene citrate.

GAMETE INTRAFALLOPIAN TRANSFER (GIFT)

In 1984, Dr. Ricardo Asch introduced a therapeutic gamete-related technique that has gained widespread popularity in the United States. It involves the injection of one or more eggs mixed with washed, capacitated, and incubated sperm directly into the fallopian tubes. Dr. Asch is believed to have come up with the acronym GIFT—*gamete intrafallopian transfer*—in order to promote the concept that GIFT gives the gift of life.

GIFT is usually done through laparoscopy. It can also be performed transcervically by the introduction of a catheter through the cervix into one of the fallopian tubes, where the sperm and eggs are discharged. Although it has yielded pregnancies in the past, this later approach has produced very disappointing results and has not gained widespread popularity. Accordingly, for all practical purposes the performance of GIFT requires laparoscopy.

The woman is usually stimulated with fertility drugs in order to achieve superovulation before the eggs are harvested for a GIFT procedure. The eggs can be removed through vaginal ultrasound-guided needle aspiration prior to administering general anesthesia or at the time of laparoscopy through the introduction of a needle via the abdominal wall. The former approach has the distinct advantage of allowing cancellation of the laparoscopy if no eggs are retrieved. The eggs are then mixed with sperm that has been previously washed and capacitated in the laboratory, and then both the eggs and sperm are loaded into a fine catheter.

If GIFT is performed during laparoscopy, the physician injects the eggs and sperm into the fallopian tubes under direct vision through the laparoscope. In this case of mini-laparotomy, the physician gently moves the ends of one or both fallopian tubes outside the abdomen through the incision, injects the sperm and eggs directly into the tubes, and then carefully returns them to the abdominal cavity before closing the abdomen.

A possible advantage that GIFT holds over intrauterine insemination is that GIFT ensures that the eggs and sperm arrive simultaneously at the point in the fallopian tubes where fertilization would normally occur. By placing the eggs and sperm together in the outer third of the fallopian tubes, GIFT eliminates any concern regarding the ability of the fimbrial ends of the fallopian tubes to pick up or receive the eggs at the time of ovulation. In effect, GIFT substitutes incubation in the body for incubation in the petri dish prior to fertilization.

Because GIFT as currently performed requires laparoscopy, it is also significantly more expensive and physically demanding than most other techniques described in this chapter. The cost of GIFT approaches that of IVF because, in addition to laparoscopy, it also requires general anesthesia.

The intensive care provided in the IVF laboratory maximizes the chances for fertilization. GIFT, in contrast, simply places a large number of sperm in the fallopian tube near an otherwise unprepared egg; hence, fertilization is much more of a hit-or-miss situation. Accordingly, we believe that GIFT, with a few exceptions, is *not a* good choice for treatment of unexplained or male infertility unless the woman requires a laparoscopy for reasons other than infertility treatment and GIFT can be performed concomitantly.

Ectopic Pregnancies with GIFT

It was initially believed that injection of the male and female gametes into the fallopian tubes during GIFT might increase the risk of ectopic pregnancies. However, statistics have not borne out this concern in cases in which the tubes are apparently normal in configuration and where no other pelvic disease is present.

A significant increase in the incidence of ectopic pregnancies has, however, been reported when GIFT is performed in women with abnormal fallopian tubes. Such pregnancies might occur even though tubal reconstructive surgery appears to have restored the patency as well as the outward appearance of fallopian tubes previously distorted by disease. Although the outward appearance of fallopian tubes may suggest they are normal, there is currently no reliable method of determining whether their internal integrity has been restored. Diagnostic procedures such as hysterosalpingogram, or injection of dye, may reveal that the tubes are open; but such examinations by no means assess whether the inner lining of the tube has been partially damaged or if the wall of the tube might be less mobile than desired.

Undetected defects in the interior of the fallopian tubes can lead to devastating consequences from GIFT. For example, damage to the interior of a fallopian tube from disease might inhibit normal physiologic function and/or peristaltic movements. Thus, the embryo might not be propelled toward the uterus in a timely manner. If nature's schedule is delayed because of sluggish peristaltic movements, the embryo might hatch in the fallopian tube and grow into its wall, thus creating an ectopic pregnancy.

Therefore, because of the risk of undiagnosed ectopic pregnancies, we firmly believe that GIFT should be reserved for cases in which there is no evidence of previous or existing tubal disease even though the tubes might appear to be normal or to have been restored to normalcy through surgery.

Pregnancy Rates with GIFT

The national birthrate reported with GIFT performed on women under 39 is about 30 percent. This statistic is comparable to that reported for IVF. Accordingly, there is little merit in advocating the performance of GIFT in preference to IVF. In addition, GIFT requires the additional performance of a laparoscopy, making it a more traumatic and often a more expensive alternative to IVF.

The low IVF success rate in women in their 40s has prompted some physicians to advocate the performance of GIFT in preference to IVF under the presumption that the natural environment of the fallopian tube would offer an improved setting for fertilization and, thus, pregnancy. This belief is erroneous.

It is important to keep in mind that GIFT does not require anywhere near the degree of sophisticated technical expertise in the laboratory that is required in IVF. Even the poorest IVF programs report satisfactory results with GIFT, while only the best IVF programs report high success rates with IVF. It should be noted that there is no evidence to support the thesis that the performance of GIFT in a woman over 40 affords a better chance of pregnancy than IVF in a good program. The results from GIFT must be viewed against this backdrop.

Finally, GIFT does not afford the opportunity to use leftover eggs (those not transferred to the fallopian tubes). In contrast, IVF permits leftover embryos to be cryopreserved.

In our opinion, it is about time for GIFT to be relegated to the history books.

ZYGOTE INTRAFALLOPIAN TRANSFER (ZIFT), OR TUBAL EMBRYO TRANSFER (TET)

Another option for achieving pregnancy in cases where infertility is unrelated to female organic pelvic disease involves the transfer of one or more fertilized eggs or embryos directly into the woman's fallopian tubes during laparoscopy. This is known as *zygote intrafallopian transfer* (ZIFT), or *tubal embryo transfer* (TET). As with routine IVF, this procedure requires an initial egg retrieval through transvaginal needle-aspiration and fertilization of the eggs in the laboratory. One or two days later, the fertilized eggs or embryos are loaded into a thin catheter and injected into the outer third of one or both fallopian tubes during laparoscopy.

In the past, proponents of ZIFT/TET argued that enabling the embryo to reach the uterus via its natural route (the fallopian tube) rather than by embryo transfer through the cervix increases the likelihood of implantation and a successful pregnancy. They also contended that ZIFT/TET would allow the embryos to travel down the fallopian tube on their own, and so reach the uterus at the appropriate stage of cleavage (about five days after transfer) when the uterus is optimally prepared, while IVF delivers an embryo directly into the uterus two or three days earlier. Accordingly, it was argued that ZIFT/TET was more advantageous, especially for the older woman, for whom IVF offers a lower success rate. This is not so.

It must be emphasized that the studies that previously reported encouraging and even superior results with ZIFT/TET were all poorly controlled. More recently, a number of well-conducted studies have confirmed that the pregnancy rate per embryo transferred with ZIFT/TET is the same as that reported for IVF. Accordingly, there is hardly any justifiable indication for the performance of ZIFT/TET in preference to IVF.

NATURAL-CYCLE IVF

Natural-cycle IVF involves accessing one and sometimes two follicles that might develop in a woman during a normal cycle for the purpose of fertilizing the eggs in vitro and transferring them to the uterus. Several advantages of this method are often cited. They include the facts that (1) the woman's cycle is not affected by fertility drugs, so she should have an optimum environment into which to place the embryos, (2) normal unstimulated-cycle IVF obviates the use of fertility drugs, and (3) the cost is considerably less than for IVF.

But an objective look at these arguments finds considerable evidence to the contrary. First, the amount of monitoring in a natural cycle significantly exceeds that which has to be done in a planned IVF cycle. The eggs must still be harvested, the sperm prepared in the laboratory, the embryo or embryos transferred; and an increased amount of blood testing is required in order to accurately monitor the woman's progress.

Therefore, it can be concluded that with the exception of the cost of fertility drugs, the performance of natural-cycle IVF does little to lower the overall cost of the procedure. The success rates from natural-cycle IVF are very much lower than from conventional IVF. Most programs doing natural-cycle IVF report no more than a 10 percent pregnancy rate per cycle with an anticipated birthrate of no more than 10–15 percent per cycle. Moreover, a woman stimulated with fertility drugs is likely to produce enough eggs so that some can be cryopreserved for later use, thus giving the couple an additional opportunity to achieve a pregnancy in a subsequent cycle; this, of course, is not an option during a natural cycle.

CHAPTER

14

THIRD-PARTY PARENTING: OTHER OPTIONS FOR COUPLES WITH INTRACTABLE INFERTILITY

For many couples who are unable to achieve pregnancy through conventional treatments, third-party parenting offers tremendous hope for success. Third-party parenting is a collective term for egg donation, embryo adoption, gestational surrogacy, donor sperm insemination, and adoption of a child. These procedures are options for the infertile couple to consider when the woman, for some reason, cannot produce healthy eggs or the proper gestational environment for a pregnancy, or when the man cannot produce healthy sperm.

Only a few years ago, women who did not have a healthy uterus and those who could not produce healthy eggs had the lowest chance of having their own baby. Now, quite paradoxically, through the advent of egg donation and IVF/surrogacy (IVF third-party parenting) these women have the greatest chance by far of conceiving, greater than with any other cause of infertility.

For some infertile women, disease and/or the onset of ovarian failure precludes their ability to produce a fertilizable egg. But if they have a healthy uterus and are otherwise able to bear a child, egg (or ovum) donation offers a realistic opportunity for pregnancy. Egg donation involves stimulating the donor with fertility drugs, retrieving the eggs from the donor, fertilizing them in the laboratory with sperm from the recipient's partner, and transferring the resulting embryos into the uterus of the recipient, who will carry the baby to term.

Some women are born without a uterus, while others undergo surgical removal of the uterus in later life. Sometimes uterine disease renders the woman incapable of bearing a child, and, in a minority of cases chronic ill health, such as severe diabetes, makes pregnancy inadvisable. For these couples, the option exists of having another woman—a third party or surrogate—bear a child for them. Surrogate parenting can be divided into two categories: classic surrogacy and IVF surrogacy.

In *classic surrogacy*, a healthy young woman (usually under 35) agrees with an infertile couple to be artificially inseminated with the male partner's sperm, carry the baby to term, and then turn the baby over to the couple shortly after birth. Classic surrogacy has brightened the lives of many desperate infertile couples, but it also brings with it many ethical, moral, and medico-legal dilemmas. There is no getting around the fact that because the classic surrogate provides both the egg and the womb, she is biologically the child's mother. This is the primary cause of surrogates' last-minute decisions not to give up the child. Who can ignore the intense media coverage that often erupts when a surrogate decides against giving up the baby to the infertile couple? Situations like this cause wrenching emotional turmoil for the parents, for the surrogate, and (sooner or later) for the child. Classic surrogacy currently is, nevertheless, still a widely employed method of surrogate parenting. Since we do not offer classic surrogacy in our programs at the present time, we will not discuss it further here.

EGG (OR OVUM) DONATION (OD)

For an ever-increasing number of infertile women, disease and/or the onset of ovarian failure precludes producing fertilizable eggs, thereby preventing them from achieving a pregnancy with their own eggs. Since the vast majority of such women are otherwise quite healthy and physically capable of bearing a child, *ovum donation* (OD) provides them with a realistic opportunity of going from infertility to parenthood.

Ovum donation is associated with definite benefits. First, in many instances, more eggs are retrieved from a young donor than would ordinarily be needed to complete a single attempt at achieving an IVF pregnancy. As a result, there are often embryos left over for cryopreservation and storage. The use of cryopreserved embryos in subsequent "frozen-embryo transfer cycles" (performed in our setting) gives such egg-donation couples another chance of having a baby following one egg harvest. If in spite of both the initial attempt and the subsequent transfer of thawed embryos the recipient does not conceive, she may schedule a new cycle of treatment.

Secondly, since eggs derived from a young woman are less likely than their older counterparts to produce chromosomally abnormal embryos, the risk of miscarriage and birth defects such as Down Syndrome is considerably reduced. Thus, there is rarely a need for amniocentesis or chorionic villus sampling in order to diagnose chromosome disorders that produce birth defects.

Ovum donation–related fresh and frozen embryo transfer cycles account for approximately 10 percent of the annual reported IVF births in the United States.

Indications for Ovum Donation

1. Advancing age (beyond 40) is by far the most common reason why American women elect to undergo ovum donation. In fact, the vast majority of ovum donation procedures performed in the United States involve embryo recipients over 40.

2. Declining or ceased ovarian function, the second most common indication for OD and one that usually ties in with age beyond 40 years. Women over 40 whose ovarian function is declining or has ceased as a result of surgery, infection, or endometriosis are good candidates, provided there is no uterine factor inhibiting implantation.

3. Failure to achieve a viable pregnancy following repeated attempts at IVF. In spite of repeatedly transferring two or more embryos to the uterus with IVF, pregnancy fails to occur. However, in such cases it is essential to first rule out factors that might be compromising healthy implantation.

4. Resistance to stimulation with fertility drugs. Despite repeated attempts, the ovaries fail to produce several eggs when stimulated with maximum doses of fertility drugs. Raised levels of FSH during first three days of the menstrual cycle might indicate a poor response to ovarian stimulation with fertility drugs.

5. Premature ovarian failure in women under 40 due to genetic cause, aneuploidy (e.g., ovarian dysgenesis or Turner's syndrome), surgical removal of the ovaries, or exposure to chemotherapy and/or excessive radiation.

6. Poor-quality eggs or embryos in spite of good-quality sperm, which is relatively common and one of the most rapidly growing indications for OD in the United States.

7. Premature menopause. Women who undergo menopause under the age of 40 and whose uterus is capable of responding to hormonal treatment are ideal candidates for OD-IVF.

8. The presence of genetic disorders that have a high likelihood of being transmitted via the woman's eggs to the offspring. Some of these disorders cannot be readily diagnosed through amniocentesis or chorionic villus sampling; in such cases, egg donation/IVF may be indicated.

9. Same-sex relationships where both partners wish to share in the parenting experience by one serving as egg provider and the other as the recipient.

How to Find a Good Ovum Donor

Use an ovum-donor agency. Ninety percent of ovum donation in the United States is done by way of soliciting the services of anonymous donors who more often than not are recruited through a state-licensed ovum-donor agency. SIRM's access to a dedicated donor agency provides a wide choice of donors for couples with diverse needs.

Recruit a donor you know or to whom you are related. In the vast majority of cases where the services of a known donor are solicited, it is usually by virtue of a private arrangement. It is less common for recipients to solicit known donors through an OD agency, although this does happen on occasion. In the United States, the decision to use a known donor is frequently based solely on the desire to reduce or eliminate the donor fee.

While the services of donors unrelated to the couple but known by them are sometimes sought, it is much more common for recipients to approach close family members in an attempt to retain as much of the family gene pool as possible.

When it comes to choosing a known donor, it is important to make sure that she was not coerced into participating. At SIRM we caution recipients who are considering having a close friend or family member serve as their designated ovum donor that in doing so, the potential always exists that the donor might become a permanent and an unwanted participant in the lives of their new family.

In the United States, embryo recipients who use known donors, while often sharing similar demographic characteristics with those who use unknown donors, tend to differ significantly from them when it comes to issues of disclosure. Recipients using anonymous donors tend to be far more open about the issue of their undergoing ovum donation and are more willing to tell others as well as inform the child about the nature of his or her conception.

Recruit an ovum donor from other sources.   We strongly discourage couples from obtaining an ovum donor from such sources as newspaper advertisements, or non-licensed organizations or individuals. This is primarily because of the risks the couple would run with no knowledge about the prospective donor's background (see "What are the criteria for a good egg donor?" below). Fortunately, this does not occur very often in the United States anymore.

Matching the Donor and Recipient

Ovum-donor agencies usually prepare rather extensive donor profiles. Some, such as the "Parenting Center" at SIRM, aside from offering direct personal and telephone-based access to both donors and recipients, also offer copious information and online services via a dedicated Web site (www.haveababy.com). Via such a Web site, for example, a recipient and her partner can, for a nominal fee, select or narrow down their selection of the most suitable ovum donors in the privacy of their home . . . and a growing number of candidates take full advantage of this service.

Interaction between the recipient(s) and the OD program may be conducted in person, by telephone, or online. Regardless, however, once the choice of a donor has been narrowed down to two or three, the recipient(s) is/are asked to forward all relevant medical records to their chosen ART physician, upon receipt of which an in-person or telephone-based detailed medical consultation will subsequently be held. Thereupon, a physical examination by the treating physician or by a designated qualified counterpart is scheduled. This entire process is overseen and facilitated by one of the OD program's nurse coordinators, who in concert with the treating physician will address all clinical, financial, and logistical issues as well as answer any questions. At the same time, the final process of donor selection and donor-recipient matching is completed.

Several examples of ovum-donor profiles can be found on SIRM's Web site (www.haveababy.com). In addition, copious written information about the potential donor is made available to the prospective recipient(s). Our toll-free number (800) 780-7437, the Web site, and the "discussion board" on the Web site should collectively provide ovum donors and embryo recipients with round-the-clock access to SIRM, a nurse coordinator, and/or a SIRM physician who can address all relevant issues.

Many recipients feel the compulsion to know or at least to have met the ovum donor so as to gain firsthand familiarity with their physical characteristics, intellect, and character.

What to Consider When Recruiting the Right Ovum Donor for You

Age.   Donor agencies (ourselves included) usually limit the age of ovum donors to under 35 years in an attempt to minimize the risk of ovarian resistance and negate the adverse influence of the biological clock on egg quality. In fact, some OD agencies go so far as to set their age limit at below 30 years.

Previous pregnancies.   No single factor instills more confidence regarding the reproductive potential of a prospective ovum donor than a history of her previously having achieved a pregnancy on her own, or of one or more recipients of embryos derived from her eggs having achieved a live birth. Moreover, such a track record makes it far more likely that such an OD will have good-quality eggs. Furthermore, the fact that an OD readily conceived on her own lessens the likelihood that she has tubal or organic infertility. However, the shortage in the supply of ovum donors makes it both impractical and unfeasible to confine donor recruitment to those women who could fulfill such stringent criteria for qualification.

It is not unheard of for a donor who subsequent to ovum donation finds herself unable to conceive on her own due to pelvic adhesions or tubal disease to blame her infertility on complications precipitated by the prior surgical egg retrieval and thereupon to embark upon legal proceedings against the ART physician and program. It should therefore come as no surprise that it provides a measurable degree of comfort to the OD program when a prospective donor is able to provide evidence of having experienced a relatively recent, trouble-free spontaneous pregnancy.

Personal/family medical history. Appropriate and careful history-taking is essential in order to identify any personal or family background that could point towards potential medical problems that might arise during or after the cycle of stimulation, and the egg retrieval. Systemic disease, known allergies to medications, hemorrhagic conditions, and mental disease are but a few significant examples. It is also extremely important to try and rule out potentially debilitating hereditary and chromosomal disorders that could affect the quality of any offspring arising out of the ovum donation.

Genetic screening. Most programs in the United States follow the American Society for Reproductive Medicine's (ASRM) recommendations and guidelines for selective genetic screening of prospective ovum donors for conditions such as sickle-cell trait or disease, thallasemia, cystic fibrosis, and Tay-Sachs disease, when medically indicated. Consultation with a geneticist is available in about 90 percent of programs. There are, however, still a significant number of OD ART programs in the United States that do not follow all ASRM guidelines.

Compatibility with recipient couple. Most recipient couples place a great deal of importance on emotional, physical, ethnic, cultural, and religious compatibility with their chosen ovum donor. In fact, they often will insist that the ovum donor's sexual orientation be heterosexual.

Psychological screening. Americans tend to place great emphasis on psychological screening of ovum donors. Since most donors are anonymous, it is incumbent upon the OD agency or ART program to determine the donor's degree of commitment as well as her motivation for deciding to provide this service. We have on occasion encountered donors who have buckled under the stress and defaulted midstream during their cycle of stimulation with gonadotropins. In one case, a donor knowingly stopped administering gonadotropins without informing anyone. She simply awaited cancellation, which was effected when follicles stopped growing and her plasma estradiol concentration failed to rise. Such concerns mandate that assessment of donor motivation and commitment is given appropriate priority.

Most recipients in the United States tend to be very much influenced by the "character" of the prospective ovum donor, believing that a flawed character is likely to be carried over genetically to the offspring. In reality, unlike certain mental illnesses such as schizophrenia or bipolar disorder, character flaws are usually neuroses and are most likely to be determined by environmental factors associated with upbringing and, accordingly, are unlikely to be genetically transmitted. Nevertheless, all donors should be subjected to counseling and screening, and should be selectively tested by a qualified psychologist; and, if necessary, they should be referred to a psychiatrist for definitive diagnosis. Selective use of tests such as the MMPI, Meyers-Briggs, and NEO-Personality Indicator help to assess for personality disorders. Significant abnormalities, once detected, should lead to the automatic disqualification of such prospective donors.

Free of substance abuse. Because of the prevalence of substance abuse in our society, we selectively call for urine and/or serum drug testing of our ovum donors.

Ovarian responsiveness. At SIRM we measure blood FSH, estradiol and, selectively, Inhibin B levels on the third day of a spontaneous menstrual cycle, and a vaginal ultrasound assessment of the number of *antral* (undeveloped, very early) ovarian follicles. We have noted an excellent correlation between such a follicle count and the number of mature eggs subsequently retrieved from the donor following ovarian stimulation with an appropriate dosage of gonadotropins. Consequently, a total antral follicle count (AFC) of less than 10 will often lead to the recommendation that the woman concerned be disqualified from serving as an ovum donor at SIRM.

Recipients must be made aware of the possibility of a suboptimal ovarian response even if all of these tests are within normal limits. Other measurable hormonal parameters include TSH, free T4, and prolactin, which if present in a high concentration can competitively bind with granulosa cell FSH receptors, reducing ovarian response to gonadotropins.

Freedom from STDs. ASRM guidelines recommend that all ovum donors be tested for sexually transmitted diseases before entering into a cycle of IVF. It is highly improbable that DNA and RNA viruses are vertically transmitted to an egg or an embryo through sexual intercourse or IVF. Nevertheless, the remote possibility as well as the legal consequences of the ovum donation process being blamed for an unrelated occurrence of disease states such as hepatitis B, C, or HIV demands that potential donors so infected be disqualified from participating in OD. In addition, evidence of prior or existing infection with chlamydia or gonorrhea introduces the possibility that the ovum donor so affected might have pelvic adhesions or even irreparably damaged fallopian tubes that might have rendered her infertile. As previously stated, such infertility, if subsequently detected, might be blamed on infection that occurred during the process of egg retrieval, exposing the caregivers to litigation. Even if an ovum donor or recipient who carries a sexually transmitted viral or bacterial agent is willing to waive all rights of legal recourse, a potential risk still exists that a subsequently affected offspring might later sue for wrongful birth.

What Can the Recipient Couple Expect to Undergo before IVF?

Procedures for the woman. The woman can expect to undergo medical evaluation (e.g., cardiovascular, hepato-renal, metabolic, anatomical reproductive) to ensure that she is able to carry a baby to term; uterine assessment (possibly hysteroscopy or FUS to identify all relevant uterine surface lesions, and ultrasound measurement of endometrial pattern and thickness around the time of normal or induced ovulation to assist in the assessment of implantation potential); infectious screening (to determine that the cervical mucus is free of infection with ureaplasma urealyticum, which along with mycoplasma can lead to early implantation failure and/or first trimester miscarriage); and selective immunologic evaluation and immunotherapy (for autoimmune disorders and associated with a high incidence of immunologic implantation failure, and thereupon selectively being prescribed therapeutic immunomodulation with heparin, steroids and/or immunoglobulin).

Procedures for the male. Sperm function is assessed by means of a comprehensive computerized semen analysis and semen cultures along with the performance of an indirect immunobead blood test for antisperm antibodies to establish a basis for selective enhancement of fertilization through micromanipulation procedures, including intra-cytoplasmic sperm injection (ICSI).

Preparation for the Ovum Donation Process

Preparation for ovum donation begins with full disclosure to all participants regarding what each step of the process involves from start to finish, as well as potential medical and psychological risks. All parties must be prepared to devote a significant amount of time to the task of full disclosure and must be willing to painstakingly address everyone's questions and concerns. An important component of full disclosure involves clear interpretation of the medical and psychological components assessed during the evaluation process. In addition, all parties are advised to seek independent legal counsel so as to avoid conflict of interest that might arise from legal advice given by the same attorney. Appropriate consent forms are then independently reviewed and signed by the donor and the recipient couple.

Most embryo recipients fully expect their chosen donor to yield a sufficient number of mature, good-quality eggs to provide enough embryos to afford a good chance of pregnancy as well as several for cryopreservation and storage. While such expectations are often met, this is not always the case. Accordingly, to minimize the trauma of unexpected and usually unavoidable disappointment, it is essential that in the process of counseling and of consummating agreements the respective parties be fully informed that the caregivers can only assure optimal intent and performance in keeping with accepted standards of care. No one can ever promise an optimal outcome. All parties should be made aware that no definitive representation can or will be made as to the number or quality of eggs and embryos that will or are likely to become available, the number of embryos that will be available for cryopreservation, or the subsequent outcome of the OD-IVF process.

The Cycle of Treatment

It is absolutely critical that both women's cycles be synchronized as closely as possible so that the endometrial lining of the recipient's uterus can be prepared for implantation of the transferred embryos. The female hormones estrogen and subsequently progesterone will be given to the recipient to prepare the endometrium. In the uncommon event of poor endometrial development, the couple is given the choice of either having the donor's eggs harvested, fertilized, and frozen for transfer to the recipient's uterus in a subsequent cycle or canceling the procedure.

The basic format used by most ovum donor programs is as follows:

1.   The recipient receives estrogen orally, by skin patches, or by injection. At SIRM we administer estradiol valerate by injection on Tuesdays and Fridays, and draw the recipient's blood on Mondays and Thursdays to measure estradiol concentrations in order to determine the subsequent hormonal dosage. She also undergoes ultrasound examinations at least once a week to evaluate the development of her uterus's endometrial lining. When the recipient is menopausal and therefore her ovaries are inactive, preparatory hormonal therapy can, in such cases, be initiated without GnRHa. For recipients with residual

ovarian function and who are therefore usually still menstruating, seven to 12 days of GnRHa therapy is required in order to achieve ovarian desensitization prior to commencing the hormone injections. The duration of GnRHa therapy is adjusted to synchronize the recipient's cycle with that of the donor. In some cases where the recipient does not ovulate or is postmenopausal, cyclicity is established through hormone replacement therapy, using sequential estrogen-progesterone therapy or the birth-control pill.

2. In order to stimulate ovulation of enough eggs to increase the chances of a viable pregnancy, the donor is treated with gonadotropins. But first, she is asked to use barrier contraception or to abstain from sexual intercourse in the cycle immediately prior to stimulation. Approximately seven days after ovulation occurs (as assessed by a BBT chart or a urine home-ovulation test kit), GnRHa is administered daily to prepare the ovaries. With the onset of menstruation approximately seven to 12 days later, the donor is given a blood test and baseline ultrasound examination to confirm that the ovaries are prepared and to exclude the presence of ovarian cysts. The decision is made then as to when gonadotropin therapy should commence. As soon as at least 50 percent of the donor's follicles have attained a mean diameter of greater than 15 mm, and at least two are 18 to 22 mm and her plasma estradiol concentration exceeds the number of follicles multiplied 125 pg/ml, she is given 10,000 units of hCG. The egg retrieval is scheduled for 34 to 36 hours later. Following the egg retrieval, the donor receives an injection with 100 mg of progesterone and is scheduled for a follow-up examination following ensuing menstruation.

3. The recipient starts receiving progesterone injections one day prior to the donor's egg retrieval and continues with daily injections until the eighth week of pregnancy or evidence of a negative outcome, whichever occurs sooner. On the day of the egg retrieval, the eggs are fertilized with the partner's sperm; and an embryo transfer is performed three or five days thereafter, depending upon whether three cleaved embryos or two expanded blastocysts are transferred. Two beta hCG pregnancy tests are performed, one each on the 11th and 13th day after egg retrieval. Hormonal replacement therapy is continued until the eighth week of pregnancy.

Approximately 12,000 to 15,000 ovum-donor cycles are performed in the United States annually, in which the vast majority of recipients are over 40 years of age with an average birthrate of 40 to 45 percent per cycle regardless of the recipient's age. In several programs of excellence, the per-cycle ovum donation birthrate exceeds 55 percent.

An optimal "soil-seed relationship" is central to successful procreation regardless of whether it occurs naturally, following ovulation induction with conventional IVF, or from IVF with ovum donation. Optimal egg/embryo quality is largely influenced by the age of the egg provider and the method of ovarian stimulation, and uterine receptivity is governed by appropriate endometrial development in response to hormonal therapy in the absence of uterine surface lesions, endometrial TH1 cytokinopathies, and ureaplasma infection. These factors, coupled with the embryo-transfer technique, impact significantly on outcome with OD-IVF. The age of the recipient plays hardly any role at all. (In the uncommon event of poor endometrial development, the couple is given the choice of either having the donor's eggs harvested, fertilized, and frozen for transfer to the recipient's uterus in a subsequent cycle or canceling the procedure.)

The miscarriage rate increases with the age of the egg provider rather than with advancing age of the recipient of embryos. Although age is associated with an increased incidence of miscarriage following natural conception, IUI, and conventional IVF, the incidence of miscarriage remains constant regardless of the age of the embryo recipient.

Emotional Aspects of Ovum Donation

The long-term quest for pregnancy is stressful at any age. After age 40 it takes on the added stress of the relentlessly ticking biological clock. Women between 40 and 43 who still have the ability to respond adequately to fertility drugs have the choice of attempting IVF with their own eggs or of using donor eggs. The choice of treatment is highly personal and should be considered in the light of the financial and emotional costs involved. The further the woman's age advances beyond 40 and/or the closer she gets to the menopause, the more likely it becomes that she would require multiple attempts at IVF to have even a reasonable chance of achieving a viable pregnancy with her own eggs.

However, after the age of 43 the adverse effect of age on a woman's egg quality so reduces the likelihood of successful IVF that ovum donation represents the most rational choice. The aspiring parents should be encouraged to carefully consider this reality. The couple must assess whether they can withstand the many possible disappointments on the road to child bearing. How important is it now that the child is genetically theirs? Is it more important to them at this point to achieve a pregnancy with donor eggs and get on with their lives? Potential parents have to answer these questions for themselves.

Financial Considerations for Ovum Donation

The fee paid to the ovum donor agency per cycle usually ranges from $5,000 to $8,000. This does not include the cost associated with psychological and clinical pretesting, fertility drugs, and donor insurance, which commonly cost between $3,000 and $7,000. The medical service costs of the IVF treatment cycle range between $8,000 and $14,000. Thus, the total out-of-pocket expenses for an ovum donor cycle in the United States range between $16,000 and $80,000, putting ovum donation outside the financial capability of most couples needing this service.

The growing cost of IVF with ovum donation has spawned a number of creative ways to try and make it more affordable. Here are a few examples:

1.   *Ovum-donor sharing.* One comprehensive fee is shared by two recipients. The down side is fewer available embryos for transfer as well as cryopreservation per recipient.

2.   *Egg bartering.* In exchange for deferment of some or all of the IVF fee, a woman undergoing conventional IVF gives some of her eggs to the clinic, which in turn provides them to a recipient patient. In our opinion, such an arrangement can be fraught with problems. For example, in the event that the woman donating some of her eggs fails to conceive while the recipient of her eggs does, it is very possible that the donor might suffer emotional despair and even go so far as to subsequently try to seek out her genetic offspring. Such action could be very damaging to her, the recipient, and the child.

3. *Financial risk-sharing.* At SIRM, we offer the "Outcome Based Plan" (OBP), which most recipient couples favor greatly. The OBP refunds up to 80 percent of set medical-service fees to qualifying IVF candidates who do not achieve a live birth after all embryos from a single egg retrieval have been transferred, whether fresh or in frozen cycles. OBP is designed to spread the risk among the providers and those women who conceive on the first attempt, so that women who need more than one try can afford to do so, and couples who do not conceive can choose and afford adoption or any other option.

Legal Considerations for Ovum Donation

The Uniform Parentage Act, which has been adopted by most states in the United States, declares that the woman who gives birth to the child will be regarded as the rightful mother. Accordingly, in most states there have not been any grounds to date for legal dispute when it comes to maternal custody of a child born through IVF with ovum donation. In a few states, such as Mississippi and Arizona, the law is less clear but nevertheless, as yet, has not been contested.

There is constant demand in the United States for the government regulation of the "egg market." At the same time, the enormous demand for ovum donation makes it highly unlikely that such practice will be outlawed at the state or federal level in the foreseeable future. A liberal attitude toward the provision of ART procreative options coupled with the widespread availability of ovum donors has created a new industry in the United States that we call "procreative tourism." This has resulted in an ever-growing number of aspiring recipients journeying to the United States for ART services in general and IVF with ovum donation specifically.

Moral-Ethical and Religious Considerations of Ovum Donation

The moral-ethical and religious implications of ovum donation are diverse and have a profound effect on cultural acceptance of this process. The view that everyone is entitled to have his or her opinion respected, provided that it does not infringe upon the rights of others, frames much of the attitude towards this process in the United States, and the extreme views on each end of the spectrum moderate the gentle central swing of the opinion pendulum.

How Old Is Too Old for Ovum Donation?

When is a woman too old to be a mother? Does the fact that women, who already outlive men, now attain an average life span of over 80 years of age entitle them to expand the limits of their reproductive performance? How does one rate the potential benefit of maturity and financial stability on child-rearing against the influence of youth, with its clear physical and temporal advantages but less-developed maturity, wisdom, experience, and, perhaps, long-term commitment to family? Does the sharing of youthful physical endeavors with youthful parents outweigh the potential benefits of exposure to greater intellectual stimulation that is more likely to occur with older parents, albeit for a potentially shorter period of time? These are some of the questions that come up when considering the justification and merits associated with parenting at an older age.

EMBRYO ADOPTION

Embryo adoption refers to the situation in which a woman receives embryos to which she and her partner have not contributed biologically. When both partners are infertile, both donor sperm and donor eggs must be used if the woman is to become pregnant. Previously, adoption of a child would have been such a couple's only option. Now, however, prenatal embryo adoption can be an alternative to adoption of a baby or child. We perform these adoptive procedures because we believe that apart from the fact that embryo adoption occurs far earlier than baby adoption, there is otherwise little difference between the two processes.

Donor embryos can come from several sources. For example, a woman who cannot produce her own eggs might choose to adopt one or more embryos from a donor and have them transferred into her uterus. An additional source of embryos would be couples who, finding they have more embryos than they wish to transfer after IVF, donate the extras to another couple.

The aspiring parents undergo a thorough clinical, psychological, and laboratory assessment prior to adopting embryos for transfer into the woman's uterus.

IVF (GESTATIONAL) SURROGACY

IVF surrogacy involves the transfer of one or more embryos derived from the woman's eggs and from sperm of her partner (or a sperm donor) into the uterus of a surrogate. In this case, the surrogate provides a host womb but does not contribute genetically to the baby. While ethical, moral, and medico-legal issues still apply, IVF surrogacy appears to have gained more social acceptance than classic surrogacy. We offer IVF surrogacy as an option in most of our programs.

Candidates for IVF Gestational Surrogacy

Candidates for IVF surrogacy can be divided into two groups: (1) women born without a uterus or who because of uterine surgery or disease are not capable of carrying a pregnancy to full term and (2) women who have been advised against undertaking a pregnancy because of systemic illnesses, such as diabetes, heart disease, hypertension, or certain malignant conditions.

As in preparation for other assisted reproductive techniques, the biological parents undergo a thorough clinical, psychological, and laboratory assessment prior to selecting a surrogate. The purpose is to exclude sexually transmitted diseases that might be carried to the surrogate at the time of embryo transfer. They are also counseled on issues faced by all IVF aspiring parents, such as the possibility of multiple births, ectopic pregnancy, and miscarriage.

All legal issues pertaining to custody and the rights of the biological parents and the surrogate should be discussed in detail and the appropriate consent forms completed following full disclosure. We recommend that the surrogate and biological parents get separate legal counsel to avoid the conflict of interest that would arise were one attorney to counsel both parties.

Selecting the Surrogate

Many infertile couples who qualify for IVF surrogate parenting solicit the assistance of empathic friends or family members to act as surrogates. Other couples seek surrogates by advertising in the media. Many couples with the necessary financial resources retain a surrogacy agency to find a suitable candidate. We direct our patients to a reputable surrogacy agency with access to many surrogates. Because the surrogate gives birth, it is rarely realistic or even possible for her to remain anonymous.

Screening the Surrogate

Once the surrogate has been selected, she will undergo thorough medical and psychological evaluations, including:

1. A cervical culture and/or DNA test to screen for infection with chlamydia, ureaplasma, gonococcus, and other infective organisms that might interfere with a successful outcome.
2. Blood tests (as appropriate) for HIV, hepatitis, and other sexually transmitted diseases. She will also have a blood test performed to ensure that she is immune to the development of rubella (German measles) and will have a variety of blood-hormone tests, such as the measurement of plasma prolactin and thyroid-stimulating hormone (TSH).

Whether recruited from an agency, family members, or through personal solicitation, the surrogate should be carefully evaluated psychologically as well as physically. This is especially important in cases where a relatively young surrogate or family member is recruited. In such cases, it is important to ensure that the surrogate has not been subjected to any pressure or coercion.

The surrogate should also be counseled on issues faced by all IVF aspiring parents, such as multiple births. She should also visit with the clinical coordinator, who will outline the exact process step by step. She should be informed that she has full right of access to the clinic staff and that her concerns will be addressed promptly at all times. And she should be aware that if pregnancy occurs, she will be referred to an obstetrician for prenatal care and delivery.

After the evaluations and counseling of both the couple and the surrogate have been completed, the three of them will meet. And once all the evaluations have been completed, the couple will select a date to begin treatment.

Follicular Stimulation and Monitoring of the Female Partner (Egg Provider)

The procedure used to stimulate the female partner of the infertile couple with fertility drugs and monitor her condition strongly resembles that used for an egg donor. In order to stimulate ovulation of enough eggs to increase the chances of a viable pregnancy, the female partner will be stimulated with gonadotropins. Approximately seven days after ovulation occurs (as assessed by a BBT chart or a urine home-ovulation test kit), GnRHa is administered daily to prepare the ovaries. With the onset of menstruation approximately seven to 12 days later, the female partner is given a blood test and baseline ultrasound examination to confirm that the ovaries are prepared and to exclude the presence of ovarian cysts. The decision is made then about when gonadotropin therapy should commence.

The female partner's first day of gonadotropin injections is referred to as cycle day 2. On cycle day 9, the program would likely begin intensive daily monitoring by means of blood hormone measurements and ultrasound examinations. Usually, one to three additional days of gonadotropin therapy will be required. Once monitoring confirms that the female partner's ovarian follicles have developed optimally, she is given an injection of the ovulatory trigger hCG. Then, in order to capture the eggs prior to ovulation, they are harvested 34–36 hours after the hCG injection by transvaginal ultrasound needle-guided aspiration.

Synchronizing the Cycles of the Surrogate and the Aspiring Mother

The surrogate will receive estrogen orally, by skin patches, or by injections, and then progesterone to help prepare her uterine lining for implantation. As with preparing the recipient for IVF/ovum donation, we use biweekly estradiol valerate injections in our programs. GnRHa is administered for a period of seven to 12 days in order to prepare the ovaries prior to administration of estradiol valerate. The duration of GnRHa therapy is adjusted to synchronize the cycle of the woman undergoing follicular stimulation with that of the surrogate. Once the prospective mother commences follicular stimulation, the surrogate will be given estradiol injections while continuing GnRHa therapy.

Building the Surrogate's Uterine Lining with Hormonal Injections

At SIRM the surrogate receives estradiol valerate injections on Tuesdays and Fridays, and her blood is drawn on Mondays and Thursdays to measure estradiol concentrations so the physician can determine the subsequent hormonal dosage. She also undergoes ultrasound examinations 10 days to two weeks after the first estradiol valerate injection to evaluate development of her uterine lining. Approximately four days prior to the expected day of embryo transfer, the recipient is given daily injections of progesterone to optimize endometrial development. In the uncommon event of poor endometrial development, the couple will be given the choice of having the aspiring mother's eggs harvested, fertilized, and frozen for transfer to a surrogate's uterus in a subsequent cycle, or canceling the procedure.

Transferring the Embryos to the Surrogate's Uterus

After the egg provider (woman partner) has undergone transvaginal ultrasound-guided egg retrieval, the eggs are fertilized and the embryos cultured as they would be for traditional IVF.

Approximately 72 to 120 hours following egg retrieval, the embryos are transferred to the surrogate's uterus. She then lies perfectly still for approximately one to two hours to enhance the chances of implantation and is then discharged from the clinic.

Management and Follow-up after the Embryo Transfer

The surrogate will be given daily progesterone injections and biweekly estradiol valerate injections and/or suppositories in order to sustain an optimal environment for implantation, and approximately 10 days after the embryo transfer will undergo a pregnancy test. A positive test indicates that implantation is taking place. In such an event, the hormone injections will be continued for an additional four to six weeks. In the interim, an ultrasound examination will be performed to definitively diagnose a clinical pregnancy. If the test is negative, all hormonal treatment is discontinued, and menstruation will ensue within three to 10 days.

If the surrogate does not conceive, the aspiring mother may have her remaining embryos frozen, to be thawed and transferred to the uterus of another woman at a later date. If in spite of both the initial attempt and subsequent transfer of thawed embryos the surrogate does not conceive, the infertile couple may schedule a new cycle of treatment.

Anticipated Success Rates with IVF Surrogacy

In the event that a viable pregnancy is confirmed by ultrasound recognition of a fetal heartbeat there is a better than 90 percent chance that the pregnancy will proceed normally to term. Once the pregnancy has progressed beyond the 12th week, the chance of a healthy baby being born is upward of 95 percent at SIRM. In our setting, we anticipate approximately a 50 percent birthrate every time embryos are transferred to a surrogate, provided the biological mother (the egg provider) is under 35 and the surrogate has a healthy uterus. The birthrate declines as the age of the egg provider advances beyond 35. It is important to note that there is no convincing evidence to suggest an increase in the incidence of spontaneous miscarriage or birth defects as a direct result of IVF surrogacy.

Toward Bioethics of IVF Surrogacy

The determination of ethical guidelines has not kept pace with the exploding growth and development in IVF. However, some leaders in the field are working together, sharing experiences and advice, in an attempt to formulate a code of ethics. We end this chapter with a suggestion made by Dr. William Andereck in a presentation called "Ethical Issues in the New Reproductive Technologies." He cited what he calls the "two-out-of-three rule" that he has applied to gestational surrogacy:

The genetic combination of the male and the female provide two of the essential elements which, along with gestation, are necessary to produce a human being. The two-out-of-three rule basically looks at these three elements: the egg, the sperm, and the gestational component. If at all possible, I recommend that at least two of these three components be contributed by the intended parents. If they can only contribute one, by all means please try not to get the other two contributed by the same person.

This is a good first step that can be applied to many of the situations discussed in this chapter.

15

ETHICAL IMPLICATIONS OF FERTILITY TECHNOLOGY

In an early version of this book, which was published in 1988, we discussed the pros and cons of using fresh vs. frozen sperm; the use of frozen sperm was considered cutting-edge technology at the time. In the edition published in 1995, we talked about such promising assisted-reproductive technology as fertilization/micromanipulation, including intracytoplasmic sperm injection (ICSI), and assisted hatching, including zona drilling. None of these techniques is discussed any longer in this chapter because, in many leading IVF centers, they have become standard procedures. This illustrates the short time span between ART development to practical implementation over the last two decades.

In previous editions we asked, "What would George Orwell have said about new fertility techniques such as cryopreserving eggs, sperm, and embryos for future use?" Now we ask, "What would George Orwell have said about gender selection and pre-implantation genetic diagnosis?"

CRYOPRESERVATION AS AN OPTION

Embryo/Blastocyst Freezing

Although we did consider embryo cryopreservation in this chapter in previous editions of this book, this is the first time that blastocyst freezing is discussed because transfer of embryos at the blastocyst stage is a relatively new approach.

There have been dramatic advances in the technology of freezing and storing human embryos for future use. At SIRM we sometimes cryopreserve embryos within 24 hours of fertilization (at the pronucleate stage), but usually we perform cryopreservation at 120 to 144 hours after fertilization, when the embryos have reached the blastocyst stage. We rarely if ever cryopreserve embryos at three days after egg retrieval any longer. The decision when to cryopreserve embryos is usually influenced by patient-specific indications and choices.

Regardless of when the freezing process is done, however, at SIRM at present most thawed embryos are transferred at the blastocyst stage. This means that pronucleate eggs are thawed and cultured for a few days, and those that attain the blastocyst stage of development are eligible for transfer to the uterus. Frozen blastocysts are thawed and then transferred a few hours later.

Approximately 10 percent of frozen blastocysts may be lost during the freeze-thaw process, as compared with 30 percent when embryos are frozen on the third day following egg retrieval. While there has been definite progress in this arena, the poor embryo freeze/thaw survival rate and lack of consistency in overall FET success rates still precludes the widespread application of this technology in the clinical arena. Available evidence suggests that the replacement of thawed embryos/blastocysts does not increase the risk of birth defects.

We believe that cryopreservation technology will continue to advance rapidly and will contribute significantly to the treatment of infertility in general and to successful IVF in particular. However, the future lies in the successful cryopreservation of human eggs.

Egg Freezing

A few normal births have been reported following the transfer into a woman's uterus of an embryo or embryos derived from IVF of a previously frozen and then thawed human egg. It is, however, technically far more difficult to cryopreserve human eggs than embryos or sperm. Egg freezing technology is still in its infancy. There is currently a far greater attrition rate during the freezing and thawing of human eggs than is the case for sperm or even human embryos. This is particularly significant because a woman capable of producing only a limited number of eggs per cycle can ill afford to lose most of them during cryopreservation. In addition, eggs are usually subjected to IVF during the same cycle of treatment in which they are retrieved, and it is unlikely that more than three or four eggs from any one couple would be left over and available for freezing after egg retrieval.

One of the reasons eggs are so much more sensitive to cryopreservation than sperm is believed to be the strikingly different composition of the two gametes. Sperm, the smallest cells in the body, is comprised of a large head containing the genetic material, and a tail. The egg, the largest human cell, is almost all ooplasm. The ooplasm contains the tiny microorganelles that nourish the fertilized egg and probably even the sperm once it has fertilized the egg.

Eggs are particularly sensitive to cryopreservation because freezing and thawing can produce two effects:

1. The fluid contained within the microorganelles in the ooplasm might expand during freezing, rupturing the microorganelles' membrane walls and thereby disrupting the metabolic processes within the egg. In contrast, the nuclear material that comprises most of each sperm appears to be relatively resistant to such damage.

2. The spindles from which chromosomes hang and that are indispensable to the exchange of genetic material during fertilization can be damaged when eggs are frozen and thawed. Spindle breakage could therefore potentially lead to an abnormal arrangement of chromosomes following fertilization.

It is important to keep in mind that nature is wisely selective. A defective egg almost certainly will not fertilize. If the embryo is defective, in the vast majority of cases it will not implant into the wall of the uterus. If the conceptus is damaged following implantation prior to the sixth to eighth week of pregnancy, the pregnancy will almost invariably abort. Nature makes a gallant attempt to maintain the integrity of the species by trying to ensure that defective gametes are incapable of fertilization, defective embryos do not implant, and imperfect concepti miscarry in the early stages of pregnancy.

Accordingly, an egg with defective ooplasm is highly unlikely to cause a problem, but the fact that spindle breakages have been observed following the thawing and fertilization of eggs has created some ambivalence on the part of many IVF specialists in regard to applying this technology in humans.

The present survival rate for embryos frozen on day 3 post ER following thawing, based solely on the observation that more than half of their cells appear to have weathered cryopreservation, is slightly greater than 70 percent and for good-quality blastocysts thawed the normal rate is closer to 90 percent. In contrast, it is three or four times less likely that an egg will survive freezing (with subsequent evidence of survival being healthy cleavage after fertilization). The development of newer methods promises to improve survival of frozen eggs. Although all this would seem to favor embryo freezing, it is possible that egg freezing, thawing, fertilization, and embryo transfer will ultimately prove to be far preferable to the use of embryos and could ultimately become standard practice in the IVF setting.

There are several theoretical advantages to cryopreserving eggs rather than embryos:

1.   *An egg is a known quantity.* It is likely to be healthy if it fertilizes and undergoes subsequent cleavage when thawed. In contrast, because the embryo is often transferred to the uterus immediately after thawing without undergoing further cleavage, one does not usually have the opportunity to observe whether it is indeed healthy at the time of transfer into the uterus. Because the embryo is further along the chain of evolution than an egg, the potential that an embryo damaged through freezing and thawing would produce an abnormal offspring is greater than that which could be anticipated from an embryo derived from a previously thawed egg.

2.   *Egg freezing skirts the ethical dilemma as to whether life in its earliest form is being manipulated.* Eggs, like sperm, are considered to be cells that do not have life potential on their own. However, some people believe that an embryo represents the earliest form of life and that

the 20 to 30 percent attrition rate of frozen-thawed embryos represents a form of abortion. However, the same argument cannot be applied to the freezing and thawing of eggs.

If one were to argue that it is unethical to freeze an egg because its chances of survival and subsequent fertilization are questionable, then it should likewise be unethical to freeze semen because many of the sperm also die during cryopreservation. In this context it might also be argued that the practice of vaginal intercourse is wasteful because only one or two, and rarely three or four, sperm might be capable of fertilizing eggs and producing offspring—and the remaining sperm would die. Thus, most people who have a religious or moral aversion to embryo freezing would be unlikely to have the same objection to the freezing of eggs.

3. *Eggs are easier than embryos to obtain.* Theoretically, women undergoing certain kinds of unrelated abdominal surgery might be willing to donate eggs. They could first be stimulated with fertility drugs and their eggs retrieved during surgery. These women could be reimbursed for donating their eggs to an egg bank or a waiting recipient, and the payment could help offset the cost of their surgery. Candidates might include women who undergo laparoscopy to have their fallopian tubes surgically occluded for the purpose of sterilization or women having hysterectomies for benign pelvic disease.

However, the largest source of eggs for ovum donation would be donors recruited through licensed agencies. This is already commonplace for the purpose of performing IVF with ovum donation. In addition, when more eggs are retrieved from a woman undergoing egg retrieval with IVF than are needed to optimize the likelihood that four to six embryos will be fertilized, the IVF couple might choose to donate or sell the surplus eggs to an egg bank or to other infertile women. We reject the sexist argument that it is immoral for women to sell their eggs while it is acceptable for men to sell their sperm.

4. *Excess frozen eggs could be used to better diagnose male infertility where the cause could not be otherwise diagnosed.* At the moment, hamster eggs and the hemi-zona test are used for diagnosis, but both have their flaws (see chapter 10). Ultimately, as we have stressed repeatedly throughout this book, a couple's fertilization potential can only be assessed through examining the ability of the sperm to fertilize healthy eggs.

It is indeed likely that the popularity of embryo freezing will ultimately be upstaged by egg freezing, but this will be some time in the future. However, embryo freezing will always have a place in the IVF setting because of the likelihood that when large numbers of eggs are fertilized in the laboratory, the couple will be left with more embryos than they or the IVF team would be willing to transfer into the woman's uterus. These excess embryos would either have to be allowed to die spontaneously or be frozen, stored, and kept available for a subsequent chance at conceiving should the initial IVF cycle be unsuccessful.

Nevertheless, we believe that, with few exceptions, egg cryopreservation would be the better option in the future if it can be safely and successfully performed. As the technology continues to develop and be refined, we expect that egg cryopreservation will provide a variety of benefits to infertile couples.

IMMATURE EGG (OOCYTE) RETRIEVAL

We believe that we could be coming to the end of the era when fertility drugs are indispensable to the removal of a sufficient number of eggs from a woman's ovaries. In the mid-1990s a group at Monash University in Melbourne, Australia, demonstrated the possibility of retrieving numerous healthy eggs from women who had not received any fertility drugs at all in advance of the egg retrieval. This procedure is known as immature oocyte (egg) retrieval. (To refresh your memory about egg growth and development, please see chapter 2, "The First Half of the Cycle.")

Within 10 to 12 days of the onset of normal menstruation, these researchers performed an ultrasound needle aspiration of the very small follicles in the woman's ovaries and removed immature eggs. These eggs were subjected to a complex process of maturation in the laboratory and then fertilized using ICSI. The resulting embryos were deposited in the woman's uterus a few days later.

This new procedure holds promise for the future. It allows potential access to a large number of healthy eggs without requiring the prior administration of fertility drugs. This is a very noble approach in view of the potential hazards and the exorbitant cost associated with the administration of fertility drugs.

Immature oocyte retrieval, once perfected, could become popular with egg donors, who would not have to submit to a regimen of fertility drugs prior to undergoing egg retrieval for the purpose of donating their eggs. There is little doubt the days of routinely using fertility drugs so as to ensure that a number of eggs can be harvested at any given egg-retrieval procedure are fast coming to an end.

SHOULD NEW FERTILITY TECHNOLOGY BE REGULATED?

In addition to the questions raised by the cryopreservation issues, new ART technology raises a host of other moral and ethical issues that have yet to be resolved—and probably never will be answered to everyone's satisfaction. The basic question is: To what extent should technology be allowed to alter the normal course of nature? In other words, where does it all end?

The following three examples illustrate the kinds of moral and ethical questions the laboratory director of a major IVF program encounters:

A 28-year-old female medical student asked:

Is it possible for you to freeze two or three stimulated cycles of my eggs now? I'll be over 35 by the time I get out of medical school, and I'd like to begin my family at about age 40, but with age-28 eggs.

When a graduate student received widespread publicity after the birth of identical twin calves from a cow embryo he had split, a couple inquired of the laboratory director:

Would you please split one of our embryos so we can have identical twins?

And a terminally ill man asked:

My wife has agreed to bear me a large family after I'm gone. Would you freeze several samples of my sperm and artificially inseminate her over the years so she could have my family?

The medical director and other key staffers of an IVF clinic should fully expect to be confronted with many such requests in the future. Although addressing these dilemmas is not within the scope of this book, the examples mentioned throughout this chapter illustrate but a few of the moral and ethical issues that arise with IVF and related technologies.

Artificially Produced Embryos

Another approach that is theoretically possible would be injecting one or more blastomeres into a zona whose contents had previously been removed or enveloping them with an artificial zona and then transferring the artificially produced embryos into a woman's uterus. It is also possible that human embryos potentially could be nurtured in the uterus of another species.

HUMAN CLONING: ARE WE GOING TOO FAR?

Following the successful cloning of an adult sheep in Scotland in 1997, scientists, theologians, physicians, legal experts, talk-show hosts, and editorial writers raised concerns about the prospect of cloning a human being. At the request of the President, the National Bioethics Advisory Commission (NBAC) held hearings and prepared a report on the religious, ethical, and legal issues surrounding human cloning. The report recommended a moratorium on efforts to clone human beings.

The term *cloning* refers to three procedures, each with very different objectives: reproductive, embryo, and biotherapeutic cloning.

Reproductive Cloning

The objective of reproductive cloning is to replicate an existing animal by removing the DNA of one of its cells and swapping it with the DNA in an egg from the same species. Following this process of "artificial fertilization," the resulting pre-embryo is either transferred directly to the uterus or is allowed to divide several times before being transferred. This procedure has been used to clone sheep and other mammals. In the process, however, serious genetic developments have been noted in more than 30 percent of the offspring. It is likely that the same attrition rate would occur in humans; and coupled with the belief that cloning disregards the sanctity of human life, reproductive cloning has caused many medical ethicists to find this procedure morally repugnant. There have been a few claims of successful cloning in humans, but none of these claims had been substantiated at the time of this writing.

Embryo Cloning

This experimental medical technique can also be referred to as "embryo splitting." It produces identical twins or triplets by replicating the process that nature uses to accomplish the same goal. In this process, the embryo is sliced in half or into thirds and allowed to develop further; and the separate sections are transferred to the uterus. The procedure is unlikely to produce an increased risk of birth defects and has the potential to enhance the likelihood of pregnancy in infertile patients who have been classified as "poor responders." The possible advantages are:

1. The potential for achieving improved IVF success with one good-quality embryo.

2. By increasing the number of transferable embryos derived per fertilization of each egg, there could be a potential to obtain acceptable IVF pregnancy/birth rates in women who because of age and/or poor response to fertility drugs are otherwise hard-pressed to produce even a single viable embryo with IVF.

Biotherapeutic Cloning

The first step in biotherapeutic cloning is the same as for reproductive cloning. The purpose of biotherapeutic cloning is to generate embryos for the purpose of research, mainly by harvesting the early embryonic stem cells that have the potential to develop into different tissue types, depending upon the environment into which they are delivered and the stimulus evoked. The production of a healthy replica of a diseased tissue or organ could be vastly superior to relying on organ transplants, and the supply would be unlimited. Theoretically, at least, there would be no risk of post-transplant organ rejection and therefore no need to use immunosuppressive drugs.

In 2004 a CNN poll found that 90 percent of Americans thought that cloning was bad, 67 percent felt that cloning animals was also a bad idea, 45 percent believed that humans will be cloned within a decade, and over half believed that human cloning is "against God's will," while 23 percent disagreed.

SOME ETHICAL CONSIDERATIONS

In the early 1980s, a plane crash cut short the lives of an infertile couple, leaving two frozen embryos orphaned. The ethical and legal questions that arose seemed endless. Did the embryos have a right to be born? If so, did they inherit the couple's estate? Who would have decision-making powers over the fate of the embryos?

Should we cryopreserve and store eggs from a young woman wishing to defer procreation until it becomes convenient? Would it be acceptable to eventually have a woman give birth to her own sister or aunt? Should we store viable ovarian tissue through generations? Should egg donation also become a future source of embryos generated for the purpose of providing stem cells to be used in the treatment of disease states or to "manufacture" fetuses as a source of spare body parts? If the answer to even some of these questions is yes, where are the checks and balances? Who will exercise control, and what form should such control take? Are we willing to engage this slippery slope where disregard for the dignity of the human embryo leads us to the point where the rights of a human being are more readily ignored? Personally, we hope not.

The answers to such questions must currently be formulated in the absence of clear ethical and legal guidelines to direct the use of IVF and related procedures. Because of this, leading professional organizations, such as the Ethics Advisory Board of the U.S. Department of Health, Education, and Welfare; the American Society for Reproductive Medicine (ASRM); the American College of Obstetricians and Gynecologists; and the Judicial Council of the American Medical Association (Ethics Advisory Board) are attempting to establish guidelines that would clarify the responsibilities of participants and set professional standards in the United States. All of the objectives dealt with by the various committees in this country and abroad are subject to a wide variety of interpretations. Furthermore, depending on demographics, geography, and the preponderance of different religious persuasions, ethical guidelines have to be modified to comply with acceptable standards within a particular community.

When one addresses the issues of morality and ethics in any particular IVF setting, it is imperative to examine not only the morality and ethics pertaining to sophisticated "Orwellian" developments in the field, such as embryo and gamete freezing, but also the "morality" of the entire technology. Examples of the kinds of questions one could ask in this regard are: Is the treatment of infertility itself justifiable? Where does one draw the line in implementing the various reproductive technologies?

In the absence of legally enforceable ethical standards of practice in the United States, each IVF program has virtually free rein with regard to the manner in which standards of ethics and morality will be applied. Largely for that reason, we work with an Ethics Advisory Board to review our ethical guidelines, to monitor our practical application of those guidelines, and to advise us in situations where difficult ethical decisions must be made.

The number of moral and ethical questions will only increase as new applications of assisted reproductive technology are introduced. Therefore, in order to answer those questions plus the ones that already confront us, we look forward to a day when clear ethical and legal guidelines directing the use of IVF and related procedures are available to everyone.

16

PUTTING THE
IVF HOUSE
IN ORDER

This book is based on the premise that IVF consumers (infertile couples and referring physicians) are at a great financial and informational disadvantage, and that the situation is not likely to change in the near future. If it is to improve at all, everyone who has an interest in IVF in the United States—physicians and others involved in IVF programs, insurance companies, fertility support groups, legislators, and IVF consumers—must work together in a concerted effort to help get the IVF house in order.

Many experts agree that there is a great need for the IVF community to deal with the consumer more openly. As far back as 1986, Dr. Gary Hodgen made the following statement at a medical conference:

I really believe that the public trust is the single greatest factor that has allowed the miracles of medicine to evolve in the twentieth century . . . The public has allowed us a great deal of latitude to decide where we are going to go and how we are going to get there. I don't believe we have in all cases returned that respect with an equal degree of explanation and understanding, speaking to the fears and concerns of the public in general. Certainly we are not of a single mind among ourselves as to the appropriate course or end-point in decision-making with regard to the ethics of in vitro fertilization therapy and research.

We believe this statement to be as true today as it was then.

How can the IVF medical community respond to that public trust? We believe the first step would be to make IVF more accessible to all consumers. IVF programs could work toward this goal by (1) cooperatively standardizing procedures so consumers can expect about the same success rates wherever they go, (2) willingly providing reliable and understandable data to consumers, and (3) working with insurance companies and legislators to make the process affordable.

A proactive approach toward compiling and disseminating IVF information on the part of the medical community would go a long way toward educating members of the media, who all too often misunderstand and consequently misrepresent what IVF is all about. We are faced with too many contentious newspaper editorials and oversimplified TV news reports that paint an inaccurate and sometimes alarming picture about the success of IVF. Reversing the harmful trend of bad press by being openly accountable is one giant step that could be undertaken immediately.

CONSUMERS HAVE THE *RIGHT* TO EXPECT MINIMUM STANDARDS IN ALL PROGRAMS

Standards must be established for IVF programs in the United States, and consumers must have easy access to understandable data about success rates. In almost all other medical disciplines, consumers can safely assume that the physician who is going to perform a certain procedure has, or has access to, the required expertise. This should be true with IVF programs as well.

Consumers deserve to have similar outcomes from every IVF program in the United States. It is unacceptable that certain programs can promise a birthrate in excess of 50 percent per treatment cycle while others report less than half this success rate—or have no track record at all on which to base any statistical analysis. Is it right that a couple should pay such a huge amount when they don't know what their chances are?

One way in which IVF programs can meet minimum standards is by learning from and replicating proven programs. The general factors that contribute to a successful IVF program can be viewed as a triangle, with each side of the triangle representing a crucial ingredient: (1) technical expertise, (2) proven clinical and laboratory protocols and techniques, and (3) rigid quality assurance. The people who make an IVF program effective constitute the glue that holds the sides of the triangle together: commitment, teamwork, and determination are essential ingredients for the successful IVF program.

The structural integrity of this triangle might be compared to the interdependence between a lock and key. Once established (i.e., the IVF program functions effectively and the key opens the lock time after time), the winning combination should not be weakened through needless, ill-conceived tinkering. In the IVF program, as in the lock-and-key example, there is zero tolerance for deviation from a successful relationship. Just as it would be silly to file away at a key that fits a lock perfectly, it is also shortsighted to refuse to take advantage of state-of-the-art technical expertise, proven protocols and techniques, and unwavering quality assurance in the IVF setting. The technology exists. Lock-and-key IVF procedures can be replicated at many sites, enabling settings that adopt them to standardize their programs and, consequently, their success rates.

The difference between a poor and an excellent IVF program may have nothing to do with availability of expertise, equipment, or technical know-how. It simply may be the way in which the components are put together. In the case of a poor program, all the components may be in place, including technical expertise, but the program may be so poorly administered that there is no uniformity of outcome. An IVF program that doesn't have any set protocols and procedures might, with luck, come up with some good outcomes over a period of time—some good results in simple cases and worse results in difficult cases, with no consistency in success rates. A consistently successful IVF program will, depending on individual requirements determined beforehand, arrange the same components differently, but the components will be the same. A consistently successful IVF program can repeat the same strategies over and over and still adopt a reliable format for cases whose special circumstances require a special approach. The only time change would be called for would be in the introduction of new technology that improves the process.

We strongly believe that there should be a way to guarantee that the components of successful IVF programs can be replicated everywhere. Consumers should be able to have confidence that no matter where they live, they will have access to a program offering the same success rates as all others. The only way to accomplish this is by ensuring that all IVF programs use practiced and proven formulas for success, and that all results are validated and available to the public. Adoption of such techniques would be a giant step forward.

CONSUMERS HAVE THE *RIGHT* TO AFFORDABLE IVF

The high cost of IVF confronts consumer, physician, and insurance company with this chicken-and-egg situation: IVF is expensive because it is a relatively new, high-tech procedure; *however,* a greater volume of IVF consumers could lower both fixed and variable costs; *but,* few customers can afford IVF because most insurance companies will not cover it; *and,* insurance companies are reluctant to reimburse for IVF because the success rates vary so widely and there is no accountability; *therefore,* IVF continues to be prohibitively expensive because . . . and the cycle continues.

The reluctance of most members of the insurance industry to cover IVF should be viewed from their perspective: They are unwilling to accept the current statistics on clinic success rates. There are many reliability problems with current statistics. There is no universal method for measuring success. Only with accurate data can insurers calculate their risk and decide on a fair premium for this kind of coverage. Then, and only then, will IVF be covered by insurance companies.

What Can Be Done to Reduce the Cost of IVF?

We believe that because fewer than 200,000 IVF procedures (out of the pool of more than 2 million potential IVF couples) are currently performed yearly in the United States, most of the more than 350 programs in this country are grossly underutilized. The number of procedures performed barely scratches the surface of the demand. One-half of all the IVF procedures in the United States are probably performed in fewer than 30 programs, with the remainder being divided among the remaining clinics. Some larger programs are doing more than 500 procedures a year, which means that others are performing far fewer than 100. Yet no one can gain optimal expertise doing so few procedures per year. It is impossible even to develop statistics, let alone confidently report them, when they are based on such small samples.

Most important, consumers must be attracted to IVF because of its reliability and quality. But merely interesting more consumers in the concept of IVF is not enough—the procedure must be made affordable, which brings us back to the issue of medical insurance coverage.

Outcome-Based Reimbursement (OBR): A New Concept of Financial Risk-Sharing with Patients

The absence of insurance coverage for IVF, with its high cost, makes it unaffordable to most who need it. Furthermore, given a 30 percent national IVF birthrate, most women will require more than two attempts to have a baby. As such, when it comes to IVF, the traditional "fee for service" system of payment puts having a baby outside the reach of the majority of infertile couples. It is against this background that SIRM introduced a new concept in payment for IVF services: Outcome-Based Reimbursement (OBR). OBR allows couples for whom IVF is medically indicated (using whichever is appropriate—their own or donor-derived eggs) a significant reimbursement for in-house clinical and laboratory-related services associated with the performance of IVF (medication and anesthesia costs excluded) if the transfer of all (fresh and frozen) embryos does not result in a live birth. Those who have a baby with the first attempt pay a premium, and the center accepts an overall reduction in fees in order to make it affordable for women who are not successful in their first attempt to be able to try several times.

OBR has met with uniform acceptance on the part of consumers. In stark contrast is the fact that most IVF physicians oppose the concept, arguing that the value of medical care is inherent in the service itself and not in the outcome. Central to this argument lies a fear that were OBR to be adopted universally for IVF services, the relatively low birthrates reported by many programs would threaten their economic survival. We submit that the absence of universal insurance coverage for IVF couples, with the high cost of IVF services, renders any such argument null and void. Rather, the challenge is to improve outcomes, not to protect the status quo.

Insurance Coverage Is the Key to IVF Affordability

During an appearance on the *Oprah Winfrey Show,* one of the authors (GS) made the following observation about the double standard that exists today with regard to insurance reimbursement for certain fertility treatments in the United States:

When most insurance companies reimburse for procedures such as penile implants done in cases of male impotence and yet refuse to cover infertility, it makes one wonder how many directors and CEOs of these companies are older men who view male impotence as a life-endangering condition and the desire of a woman to have a baby as a vanity.

This double standard also applies to reimbursement for tubal surgery (see "Comparing Apples and Oranges—Tubal Surgery vs. IVF," in chapter 9). Until insurance companies change their outlook, this double standard will be perpetuated.

Before insurance companies are likely to cooperate, IVF programs must openly account for their success rates. All United States IVF programs should submit their statistics on quality of service for review by an impartial accrediting agency.

Why Insurance Companies Are Reluctant to Cover IVF—And What It Will Take to Fix It!

In the United States, one of the richest and most technically advanced nations on earth, millions of couples remain involuntarily childless. A conservative estimate places the number of U.S. couples that grapple with infertility annually at 5 million, yet less than 20 percent of those couples will undergo some form of definitive treatment. The high cost of infertility treatment, especially IVF, has resulted in reluctance on the part of most insurance companies to provide benefits for infertility and, therefore, has rendered such medical intervention financially inaccessible to the general infertile population. Although a few states have enacted legislation requiring health insurance providers to offer or provide infertility benefits, such coverage is often limited or absent altogether due to regulatory loopholes. The majority of employer groups as well as health insurance providers continue to avoid voluntarily including infertility benefits. They recognize that such benefits would spawn an increase in the demand for these specialized services. This fuels their fear of the spiraling costs that might be brought about by a disproportionate increase in the demand for expensive ART and the costly neonatal services required to deal with the potential influx of premature babies resulting from IVF-related multiple births.

These facts notwithstanding, it is inevitable that the strong and rising tide of consumer demand in response to compelling scientific evidence in support of IVF and other non-experimental ARTs as valid treatment options will ultimately force a much-needed change. It is our contention that unless medical and insurance providers abandon the existing stalemate and work together to reach agreement that leads to the rapid introduction of voluntary, universal insurance benefits for infertility, including ART, there will occur a rising tide of consumer discontent that will become a catalyst for a government-imposed resolution. It would be preferable by far for medical and insurance providers to commit to working in unison to resolve this problem rather than having heavy-handed bureaucratic legislation thrust upon us. The development of a strategy that would enable insurance providers to control costs and quality by monitoring utilization and treatment outcome, while discouraging abuses of the system, could put voluntary universal infertility insurance coverage well within reach.

Historically, the insurance industry has resisted the provision of voluntary infertility benefits on the basis of the following:

1. Lack of accountability in reporting of ART/IVF success rates
2. Fear of precipitating adverse enrollee selection

3. The significant incidence of high-order multiple births (triplet pregnancies or greater) and the associated medical costs and social consequences

4. Significant disparity in success rates among ART programs.

Lack of accountability in reporting IVF success rates. The field of ART, which involves IVF and related procedures, has repeatedly been the focus of heated debate and controversy. Is this due to the fact that this area of medicine that deals with the initiation of life is regarded as sacrosanct, or is it because the practice of ART is so prone to misrepresentation and lack of accountability that it is regarded by many as fraudulent? Why is it that a couple researching their chances of undergoing successful IVF in two different ART clinics in the United States will often find that the live birth rate in one center is two to three times higher than in the other? And why, with a reported national average birth rate for IVF in women under age 39, using their own eggs, of about 30 percent per egg-retrieval procedure, do these couples encounter outcome statistics that range from single digits in allegedly poor programs to more than 50 percent in better ones?

Even worse, why, when turning to professional medical oversight bodies such as the Society for Assisted Reproductive Technology (SART) and the Centers for Disease Control (CDC) to answer these questions and help them identify and select an IVF program on the basis of its proven track record, do consumers find themselves stonewalled? Because there is currently no verifiable system of outcome-based IVF reporting in America. Furthermore, the current practice by SART of reporting conventional IVF statistics under a single broad category—the woman's age—is of little value to the individual IVF candidate. The multitude of variables that influence IVF outcome renders any attempt at interpreting IVF outcome based upon such a broad generalization misleading, and possibly even deceptive. Despite sixteen years of repeated promises to implement verifiable reporting of clinic-specific IVF success rates, SART's current system of "quality assurance" falls far short of achieving this objective, and as such, does not protect the consumer from manipulation.

The current criteria for clinic-specific reporting by SART-member programs are unenforceable. For the most part, the SART report consists of self-generated data submitted by ART programs and published unaudited and/or unvalidated, largely upon the basis of "good faith." In the virtual absence of oversight and accountability, it is a relatively simple matter for any IVF program to overstate their number of IVF "successes," understate their number of "failures," and/or "improve" their success rates by selectively performing IVF on only those cases most likely to succeed (e.g., younger women, women with few or no prior IVF failures, and women who, based upon testing, are most likely to respond optimally to fertility drugs). Given that the practice of IVF in the United States is highly competitive and consumers understandably prefer to undergo treatment at the most successful centers, it should come as no surprise that with little or no risk of being detected and minimal consequences if they are, some IVF programs do indeed overstate their success rates.

A historical perspective may provide further insight. SART was originally established in New Orleans at the annual meeting of the American Fertility Society in 1984. At that time it was named the "IVF Special Interest Group." For several years it was the policy of the IVF Special Interest Group to annually report only pooled data (i.e., the collective results of its entire ART-program membership). In fact, each member program that submitted its annual statistics for inclusion in what was then known as the IVF Registry was given assurance by the custodians of the Registry that only pooled data would be made public. Further, Registry members were actually advised *not* to disclose their clinic-specific outcome data based upon the belief that it would make it less likely that IVF programs would overstate their success rates in order to be competitive.

In 1986, prompted by numerous complaints regarding exploitation and unscrupulous practices in the arena of infertility in general and IVF in particular, the United States Congress took action. Hearings were held under the auspices of the Office of Technology Assessment (OTA) to address consumer concerns. In 1989 the proceedings and the conclusions were published in the "Wyden Report." Congress subsequently mandated, under threat of prosecution, that all IVF programs in the United States report their outcome statistics for 1987; and as a result, the first report of clinic-specific ART outcome statistics in the United States was published. This was followed by passage of the "IVF Success Rate Certification Act of 1992," which was implemented in 1997. The explicit intent of this act was to compel honest disclosure of IVF success rates and the implementation of quality assurance in all IVF programs in the United States.

In 1994, sensing a growing consternation among IVF consumers regarding its continued nonaccountability, SART gave tacit support to the introduction of an "audit" of all its member programs. The national accounting firm of Peat Marwick & Company was engaged to develop and help implement a clinic-specific, IVF-outcome-based reporting process. Disinterest on the part of ART centers, coupled with SART's lack of resolve to enforce compliance, resulted in this attempt at a verification process being abandoned before the year ended. Perhaps not unexpectedly, subsequent gestures on the part of SART to introduce alternate methods for the appropriate verification of IVF outcome reporting have led to nothing more than the virtual "self-reporting process" that currently exists, and which is supported by "token" random and sporadically conducted on-site reviews. The ultimate complete failure of this process became self-evident in July 2002, when SART sent a letter to all IVF program directors in the United States stating that as a result of a "lack of financial and human resources," random on-site reviews would be foregone with respect to outcome data for the year 2000. Instead, SART directed all medical directors of its member programs to perform a specified "self-review" of the medical and laboratory records of ten pre-selected IVF cases. Upon receipt of such information in the required format, the center would pass certification and thereupon would undertake to publish the program's total, self-generated IVF outcome data for the year 2000 on the Centers for Disease Control's (CDC's) official Web site.

As long as SART refuses to demonstrate a commitment to fulfill their obligation to assure honesty in reporting of IVF outcome data, the insurance industry will likely remain skeptical and reluctant to pay for IVF.

Fear of adverse enrollee selection.   There is concern on the part of individual insurance companies and employer groups that a decision to provide benefits for ART would cause infertile couples to take rapid, excessive, and possibly ill-advised advantage of the coverage and ultimately result in an unreasonable financial liability. The implementation of a reporting system based on outcome (the Outcome Based Reporting, or OBR, see above) will work to avoid these concerns. It will minimize risks to insurance companies and actually help them to enroll otherwise healthy families, who, it is anticipated, will become loyal members for a substantial period of time into the future.

High incidence of IVF-related multiple births.   In an attempt to optimize success rates, many IVF programs in the United States still transfer relatively high numbers of embryos with the hope that at least one will result in a pregnancy. The result has been an unacceptable increase in the incidence of high-order multiple births. High-order multiple pregnancies, because they compound the incidence and severity of most pregnancy-induced complications and are associated with a high risk of premature delivery, are prejudicial to the health of both the mother and her offspring. Premature birth leads to a high perinatal mortality and morbidity with complications that can prevail throughout the life of the offspring. Such prematurity-related, life-long morbidity establishes an enormous potential financial burden for insurance providers and thus creates a strong disincentive to provide benefits for ART services. Although the ASRM has published guidelines relating to the numbers of embryos to be transferred to a given patient, there is currently no reasonable method to mandate the maximum number of embryos that may be transferred. Consequently, the insurers have no control over this variable. This problem can only be solved through penalizing IVF providers whenever a high-order multiple pregnancy occurs as the direct consequence of transferring an inappropriately high number of embryos.

Disparity in IVF success rates.   The wide disparity in IVF success rates reported by ART programs in the United States has understandably led providers of health insurance to question and investigate the varying levels of expertise with respect to these services. This disparity in IVF success rates, coupled with an awareness that there is currently no way of accurately verifying reported success rates, has eroded confidence in the entire ART industry and has contributed to reluctance on the part of insurance companies to fund such services.

In those states that mandate IVF coverage, leaving insurance payers with little choice but to comply, costs have spiraled out of control and have led to a progressive reduction in the reimbursement for IVF services. ART programs have been forced to respond by increasing their productivity in order to remain profitable. To achieve this, many physicians had "cut corners" by involving more paramedical and/or technical personnel in the performance of procedures that they themselves would ordinarily do (e.g., such as ultrasound monitoring of follicle growth) and by devoting less time to the individual patient. Predictably, such actions have led to a decline in the standard of care and reduced IVF success rates.

The time has come for an immediate commitment to solve this problem. The formulation of a strategy must include development of a verification process that would permit real monitoring of IVF utilization and outcome, one that rewards for good performance in terms of outcome in well-defined categories of clinical complexity (so as to allow outcome to be evaluated in comparable patients), discourages and penalizes abuses of the system, including but not limited to the reckless transfer of large numbers of embryos, and does all this in real time, providing easy access of results to all interested parties (consumers, governing bodies, and insurance providers).

If this is done, universal IVF insurance coverage could well become within reach, since there could be a significant financial upside for insurance companies, through tapping into the large infertility community. After all, aside from reproductive problems, the infertile population in the United States is relatively young and healthy, comprised of individuals who are less likely to require costly medical care and whose need to keep their insurance coverage current at all times would likely ensure their fiscal responsibility. Moreover, employers could offer access to infertility coverage as an added benefit by which they could attract high-quality employees.

Some Novel Approaches

The first step towards attaining the worthy objective of universal infertility coverage requires introduction of a method that will allow for reliable verification of clinic-specific outcome data (birth rates per cycle of treatment) for every possible demographic category. A computerized data collection system could be placed in every participating ART program, with the requirement that only those procedures that are fully entered within 72 hours of completion would be eligible for insurance reimbursement. This would permit accurate and verifiable outcome reporting along with oversight relative to the number of eggs/embryos being transferred. All ART programs could be required to meet specific performance standards in order to qualify for insurance reimbursement and be rewarded with financial incentives if performance exceeded required standards. In this way, by shifting the focus from service to outcome, there would evolve a strong incentive to upgrade standards of care, improve outcomes, and minimize the number of treatment cycles necessary to achieve a live birth.

It is imperative that health insurance providers be embraced as part of the solution rather than being regarded as part of the problem. An all-inclusive multi-institutional "think tank," made up of physicians, consumers, and insurance providers, should be convened without delay to discuss the feasibility of introducing universal infertility insurance coverage in the United States. It is time to take the cause for optimal, safe, and affordable infertility care to the ones who need it the most—the consumers. The overriding goal must be to have the insurance industry join all interested parties in the immediate establishment and enforcement of a workable regulatory process.

Change is sometimes difficult to accept and implement. We anticipate that these novel approaches will create anxieties and objections from established, albeit outdated and inadequate, data-collection programs such as the ones currently in place and overseen by SART and the CDC. But we believe that the approaches outlined above would create necessary checks and balances to provide cost-effective, voluntary, universal insurance benefits for advanced ARTs, with widespread and far-reaching advantages for the employer, the pharmaceutical companies, the physicians, and—above all—prospective and existing patients.

We have to make a start . . . and there is no time like the present.

IVF CONSUMERS HAVE AN *OBLIGATION* TO GET INVOLVED

Ultimately, consumers can control the debate. They may have to band together to make their voices heard against the forces of the marketplace, but they can bring about change. Now is the time for IVF consumers to be outspoken. If they do not participate in the campaign to put the IVF house in order, they have only themselves to blame if progress comes slowly. One of the most promising lobbying avenues would be to join one of the infertility support groups, both to become more informed and to speak with a louder voice before the medical profession, legislative groups, and the insurance industry.

It is time for consumers to marshal their buying power to demand that the "big A's" in the field of high-tech infertility management, outlined in the previous section, are met:

1. Accreditation of IVF programs
2. Accountability by the medical profession with regard to providing validated and verifiable statistics or a track record, and instilling rational expectations in infertile couples who seek their advice
3. Availability and access to the consumer of state-of-the-art standards of care
4. Affordability

WHERE DO WE GO FROM HERE?

After an initial shakeout period following accreditation, the United States may have fewer IVF programs, but they will be programs validated by peer review and offering a uniformly reliable success rate. Just because there are fewer programs, however, does not mean that access to IVF will be more restricted than it is now for consumers who do not live in metropolitan areas. On the contrary, mobile units could bring

IVF and related procedures to the couple's own area, where they are familiar with the doctor and feel most comfortable.

For example, instead of 25 small programs in one geographical area, all of which have relatively high costs because they cannot benefit from economies of scale, consolidation and regionalization might provide better service to the entire area. A few large, well-equipped centers could serve outlying communities as well as the metropolitan area, reducing overhead costs while maintaining an optimal level of technology and research.

THE BOTTOM LINE

Ultimately, society itself must determine whether technology should be allowed to run rampant or allowed to progress in a controlled manner. We recognize the widespread concern of the medical community that regulation of one aspect of medicine may lead to creeping regulation of the entire profession. Nevertheless, we believe it would be socially responsible to adopt, at the national level, directives or requirements that would control this developing technology for the public good.

The social responsibility that confronts practitioners of IVF and related technologies was underscored by Dr. Gary Hodgen about two decades ago at an IVF conference in Reno when he asked:

How can we in the area of in vitro fertilization do anything other than search and struggle together to find what this moral and ethical obligation is, define it, and attempt to refine it as we move forward with research results, technology, and new capabilities to help infertile couples? There is little difference of opinion in this pluralistic society about the needs of people to have well children. The issue that's at risk is how we get there.

The time has come to move from recommendations and guidelines, inconsistently applied, to strong directives that can be enforced. Loosely stated guidelines do not provide enough direction, and they leave the field wide open to abuse. All too often, guidelines have been adopted because decision makers are afraid to say "This is what you will do" and thus settle for "This is what we recommend you might do—if you want to."

Decisions about the future directions of fertility technology cannot be left to one interest group. In our pluralistic society, varying viewpoints and backgrounds must be represented in order to make the consensus process work: consumers, physicians and other practitioners of IVF, the clergy, fertility support groups, lawyers, insurance carriers, ethics specialists, the media, and legislators must all work together to bring about the national adoption of comprehensive, enforceable directives to guide the implementation of research and clinical care in the field of infertility.

For the thousands of couples whose lives have been enriched by the gift of life through IVF and the other assisted reproductive technologies, for the many more infertile couples who have little hope of conceiving without the assistance of these procedures, and mindful of the sacred doctrine that obliges the medical profession to improve the human condition and alleviate suffering wherever possible, we challenge consumers, the medical/scientific communities, and the insurance industry to strive together to expand the technology, improve the quality, and promote the affordability and accessibility of IVF and related technologies.

GLOSSARY

A/ACP *See* agonist/antagonist conversion protocols.

acid tyrodes digestion A form of assisted hatching in which the embryo is introduced into a chemical solution that partially erodes the zona (egg covering) in order to promote hatching.

acrosome The protective structure around the head of the sperm. The acrosome contains enzymes that enable the sperm to penetrate the egg.

acrosome reaction The second stage of capacitation, when a sperm sheds its outer membrane to expose receptors that interact with the egg's zona pellucida to initiate fertilization.

adenomyosis A condition in which the endometrial glands grow into the uterine wall, creating a spongelike effect; can be associated with poor uterine linings. Women with this condition may experience heavy, painful periods and uterine enlargement.

adrenal glands Small structures located at the top of each kidney that produce a number of hormones indispensable to proper growth, development, and a wide variety of physiologic functions.

AF *See* assisted fertilization.

AFC *See* antral follicle count.

agonist/antagonist conversion protocols (A/ACP) Administration of GnRH agonist for approximately five days prior to menstruation, at which point the agonist is discontinued and a GnRH antagonist is administered daily until the hCG trigger. Simultaneous with GnRH antagonist administration, the woman receives gonadotropins daily until the hCG trigger.

AID   *See* artificial insemination by donor.

AIDS   Acquired immunodeficiency syndrome, sexually transmitted disease believed to be caused by one or a variety of viruses that are harbored in the nuclei of cells and attack the immune system. Infected individuals become highly susceptible to opportunistic infections; AIDS ultimately leads to death.

alloimmunity   Immunity that develops against the proteins of another individual of the same species.

alpha fetoprotein   A chemical in the blood and amniotic fluid that if found might point toward a neurologic fetal malformation.

American Fertility Society   Former name of the American Society for Reproductive Medicine (ASRM).

American Society for Reproductive Medicine (ASRM)   A professional society that primarily includes physicians but also includes laboratory personnel, psychologists, nurses, and other paramedical personnel interested in infertility. Formerly known as the American Fertility Society.

androgens   Male hormones produced by excessive LH that directly stimulate the tissue surrounding the ovarian follicles; some of these androgens may filter into the surrounding follicles and adversely affect both follicle and egg development.

aneuploidy   Structural and numerical chromosomal abnormalities of the egg.

antibodies to sperm   Substances in the man's or woman's blood and in reproductive secretions (semen, uterine and tubal secretions, and cervical mucus) that reduce fertility by causing sperm to stick together, coating their surface or killing them.

antilymphocyte antibodies (ALA)   Antibodies formed to combat the male partner's lymphocytes, hence also combat those of the fetus.

antiphospholipid antibodies (APA)   Antibodies to some of the chemical substances that coat the root system of the placenta as it grows into the uterine wall. Women with high concentrations of these substances may have a higher incidence of miscarriages or may fail to conceive after repeated attempts.

antral follicle count (AFC)   An ultrasound examination of the ovaries during the first few days of the menstrual cycle that reveals the presence of small antral (fluid-filled) follicles, the number of which suggests the potential number of eggs that could become available for egg retrieval under optimal stimulation.

anus   Excretory opening of the intestinal tract.

ART   *See* assisted reproductive technology.

artificial insemination by donor (AID)   The most common form of insemination into the vagina or uterus; AID involves the use of donor semen or sperm in cases where the woman's partner is infertile or the woman chooses to conceive without having intercourse with the sperm provider.

ASRM   *See* American Society for Reproductive Medicine.

assisted fertilization (AF)   Methods for promoting successful IVF in cases of severe male infertility; these approaches require highly sophisticated technical expertise and equipment. Also known as micromanipulation.

assisted hatching   A technique in which the zona pellucida (outer shell of the egg) is chemically or mechanically thinned prior to embryo transfer in order to improve the likelihood of subsequent hatching.

assisted reproductive technology (ART)   Procedures involving retrieval of eggs and the enhancement of eggs and sperm outside the body. Includes procedures such as gamete intrafallopian transfer (GIFT), in vitro fertilization (IVF), and zygote intrafallopian transfer (ZIFT)/tubal embryo transfer (TET).

augmented laparoscopy   A procedure in which eggs are retrieved from the woman's ovaries while diagnostic laparoscopy is being performed to evaluate the integrity of her pelvic organs. These eggs are subsequently fertilized in vitro, and the embryos are then transferred into the woman's uterus. This procedure affords a woman undergoing routine diagnostic laparoscopy a chance to determine the cause of her infertility and an opportunity to conceive by IVF at the same time.

autoantibodies   Antibodies that are formed against the proteins of the individual's own body.

basal body temperature (BBT) chart   A daily body temperature chart that provides a rough idea of when ovulation occurred. This is possible because body temperature rises when the corpus luteum produces progesterone (after ovulation) and drops at or just before the beginning of menstruation, when estrogen and progesterone levels fall (*see also* biphasic pattern of temperature on BBT chart).

BBT chart   *See* basal body temperature chart.

Billings Method of contraception   A method of predicting ovulation in which the woman examines the quality and quantity of her cervical mucus secretions. This method can be used to help the woman determine her most fertile period for the purpose of conceiving or for contraception.

biotherapeutic cloning   Replication of an existing animal by swapping its DNA with the DNA in an egg from the same species for the purpose of generating embryos for research purposes (e.g., stem cells).

biphasic pattern of temperature on BBT chart   Charting pattern that occurs because the woman's temperature is likely to be 0.5°F to 1°F lower during the first phase of her menstrual cycle than during the second half, when the progesterone produced by the corpus luteum raises her temperature slightly (*see also* basal body temperature chart).

bladder   The anatomical reservoir that receives urine produced by the kidneys.

blastocyst   An advanced stage of embryo development during which a cavity develops within the young embryo.

blastocyst transfer   The process of culturing embryos until they reach the blastocyst stage before transferring them to the uterus; the transfer of good-quality blastocysts is associated with a higher pregnancy rate than transfer of embryos on day 3 after fertilization.

blastomere   Cell within the developing embryo. Each blastomere is capable of developing into an identical embryo until the embryo reaches about the 30-cell stage, after which the cells begin to differentiate into specific tissues.

blastomere biopsy   Biopsy of a blastomere at the seven- to eight-cell stage of cleavage (day 3 after fertilization) for the purpose of diagnosing aneuploidies.

"blocking antibodies"   *See* antilymphocyte antibodies.

blood-hormone test (LH) When this test is performed several times daily around the presumed time of ovulation, the detection of a rapidly rising blood LH (luteinizing hormone) concentration can accurately determine the time of probable ovulation. This test, which requires blood to be drawn several times and is therefore painful, time-consuming, and expensive, has been virtually supplanted by serial urine LH testing (*see also* urine ovulation test).

blood-hormone test (progesterone) Measuring of the concentration of progesterone in the woman's blood during the second half of the menstrual cycle about one week prior to anticipated menstruation; indicates whether or not she is likely to have ovulated because progesterone is usually produced only by the corpus luteum, which develops after ovulation.

capacitation The process by which sperm are prepared for fertilization as they pass through the woman's reproductive tract (in vivo capacitation); sperm may also be capacitated in the laboratory (in vitro capacitation).

cervical canal The connection between the outer cervical opening and the uterine cavity.

cervical mucus Mucus produced by glands in the cervical canal; it plays an important role in transporting sperm into the uterus and in initiating capacitation.

cervical mucus insufficiency A condition in which the ability of the cervical mucus to initiate the capacitation process is compromised through a deficiency in the amount of mucus produced, an abnormality in the physical-chemical components of the mucus, the presence of infection, an abnormal hormonal environment, or the secretion of antibodies to sperm in the mucus. Cervical mucus insufficiency is responsible for about 10 percent of all cases of infertility.

cervicitis Inflammation of the cervix due to ureaplasma, chlamydia, or other organisms.

cervix Lowermost part of the uterus, which protrudes like a bottleneck into the upper vagina; the cervix opens into the uterus through the narrow cervical canal.

chemical pregnancy   Biochemical evidence of a possible developing pregnancy based on a positive blood or urine pregnancy test; at this point, pregnancy is presumptive until confirmed by ultrasound (*see also* clinical pregnancy).

chlamydia   Bacteria responsible for a sexually transmitted infection that may damage the fallopian tubes and/or the male reproductive ducts, thereby causing infertility.

chromosomes   Structures in the nuclei of cells, such as the egg and sperm, on which the hereditary or genetic material is arrayed.

classic surrogacy   The use of a third party to conceive and carry a baby to term. In this form of surrogacy, the baby would bear the genetic imprint of the surrogate and of the sperm provider.

cleavage   The process of cell division.

climacteric   The hormonal change that precedes the menopause by a number of years and is associated with a progressive loss of fertility, an increased incidence of abnormal or absent ovulation, hot flashes, irregular menstruation, a progressive rise in blood FSH levels, and mood changes. The climacteric usually represents an important stage in a woman's life.

clinical pregnancy   A pregnancy that has been confirmed by ultrasonic examination or through pathologic assessment of a surgical specimen obtained either from a miscarriage or from an ectopic pregnancy. A clinical pregnancy should be distinguished from a chemical pregnancy, which through a positive blood pregnancy test merely suggests the possibility that a pregnancy has occurred (*see also* chemical pregnancy).

clitoris   The small structure at the junction of the labia minora in front of the vulva. The clitoris, which is analogous to the penis in the male, undergoes erection during erotic stimulation and plays an important role in orgasm.

clomiphene citrate   A synthetic hormone that is used alone or in combination with other fertility drugs to induce the ovulation of more than one egg. When marketed in the United States, clomiphene citrate is also known as Clomid or Serophene.

COH   *See* controlled ovarian hyperstimulation.

computerized genetic hybridization (CGH)   A new technique that involves the simultaneous evaluation of all chromosomes.

conception   Creation of a zygote by the fertilization of an egg by a sperm.

conceptus   A term used to describe the developing implanted embryo and/or early fetus.

controlled ovarian hyperstimulation (COH)   In response to the administration of fertility drugs, the maturation of several follicles simultaneously, which results in the production of an exaggerated hormonal response.

corona radiata   *See* cumulus granulosa.

corpus luteum   A term for a follicle after an egg has been extruded. After ovulation, the follicle collapses, turns yellow, and is transformed biochemically and hormonally. The corpus luteum produces progesterone and estrogen, and has a life span of about 10 to 14 days, after which it dies unless a pregnancy occurs. If the woman becomes pregnant, the life span of the corpus luteum is prolonged for many weeks. A synonym for the corpus luteum is the "yellow body."

cryopreservation   The process of freezing (in liquid nitrogen) and storing eggs, sperm, and embryos for future use.

cul-de-sac   The area of the woman's abdominal cavity behind the lower part of the uterus.

cumulative birthrate   The overall chance of a woman having one or more babies per egg retrieval or per embryo transfer following several attempts.

cumulative pregnancy rate   The overall chance of a clinical pregnancy occurring per egg retrieval or per embryo transfer following several successive procedures.

cumulus granulosa   The group of ovarian cells resembling a sunburst that surrounds the zona pellucida of the human egg; also called the corona radiata. These cells nurture the egg while in the fallopian tube.

DES (diethylstilbestrol)   A drug previously taken by women during pregnancy that may cause infertility and/or pathologic conditions in the reproductive tracts of both male and female offspring.

DFI   *See* DNA fragmentation index.

diagnostic hysteroscopy   A procedure that can be performed under anesthesia in the outpatient or hospital setting with minimal discomfort for the patient. A thin telescopelike instrument is inserted via the vagina and cervix into the uterine cavity, and carbon dioxide gas or a liquid is injected to distend the cavity and allow direct visualization of its structure.

diagnostic IVF   The performance of in vitro fertilization for the purpose of assessing the ability for fertilization to take place. It is an objective test of sperm/egg fertilization potential.

DNA fragmentation index (DFI)   Numerical form in which DNA damage in sperm is expressed after the sperm DNA integrity assay.

dysmature   Condition of an egg unlikely to develop into a viable embryo capable of initiating a healthy implantation and pregnancy.

E2   *See* estradiol.

ectopic pregnancy   A pregnancy that occurs when the embryo implants in a location other than the uterus; the most likely site for such implantation is the fallopian tube (in which case the term *ectopic pregnancy* is used synonymously with the term *tubal pregnancy*). If undetected, an ectopic pregnancy may rupture and cause life-threatening internal bleeding. Ectopic pregnancies almost always require surgical intervention.

egg   The female gamete, which develops in the ovary; also known as an ovum or oocyte. An egg is the largest cell in the human body.

egg retrieval   The retrieval of eggs from the ovarian follicles prior to ovulation; the eggs are sucked out of the follicles through a needle during ultrasound guidance or, rarely, laparoscopy.

ejaculation   The emission of semen through the urethra and penis that follows erotic stimulation and accompanies male orgasm.

embryo   The term for a fertilized egg from the time of initial cell division through the first six to eight weeks of gestation. Thereafter, the embryo begins to differentiate and take on a human organic form; at this point it is traditionally referred to as a fetus.

embryo adoption   This occurs when a woman receives into her uterus an embryo to which neither she nor her partner has contributed a gamete.

embryo cloning An experimental medical technique that produces identical twins or triplets by slicing an embryo in half or into thirds and allowing them to develop further before transfer into the uterus; also known as "embryo splitting."

embryo co-culturing The addition of cells derived from the growth of other tissue (from the lining of human or bovine fallopian tubes, or human follicular lining) to the culture medium in which the zygote is being nurtured in the laboratory. This is thought to enhance growth and promote the development of healthier embryos.

Embryo Marker Expression Test (EMET) The measuring of a genetic marker known as soluble human leukocyte antigen-G (sHLA-G), which is released into the media in which early embryos are growing after fertilization, in order to identify those embryos most likely to produce a pregnancy.

embryo splitting *See* embryo cloning.

embryo transfer The process whereby embryos that have been grown in the petri dish are transferred into the uterus.

EMET *See* Embryo Marker Expression Test.

endometrial biopsy Surgical removal of a specimen of the endometrium, commonly performed to permit microscopic examination of the effect of estrogen and progesterone on the endometrium. When performed by an expert, it is usually possible to pinpoint almost to the day when ovulation is likely to have occurred.

endometrioma A cystic collection of altered menstrual blood in the ovary that interferes with optimal follicle/egg development.

endometriosis A condition in which the endometrium grows outside the uterus, causing scarring, pain, and heavy bleeding, and often damaging the fallopian tubes and ovaries in the process. Endometriosis is a common organic cause of infertility.

endometrium The lining of the uterus, which grows during the menstrual cycle under the influence of estrogen and progesterone. The endometrium grows in anticipation of nurturing an implanting embryo in the event of a pregnancy; it sloughs off in the form of menstruation if implantation does not occur.

endosalpinx   Inner lining of the fallopian tubes.

epididymis   Tubular reservoir that contains and transfers sperm to the vas deferens and subsequently through the urethra and penis at the time of ejaculation.

estradiol (E2)   A female hormone produced by ovarian follicles. The concentration of estrogen in the woman's blood is often measured to determine the degree of her response to controlled ovarian hyper-stimulation with fertility drugs. In general, the higher the estradiol response, the more follicles are likely to be developing and, accordingly, the more eggs are likely to be retrieved.

estradiol valerate   A preparation of natural estradiol taken orally or by injection.

estrogen   A primary female sex hormone, produced by the ovaries, placenta, and adrenal glands.

exit interview   An interview prior to the couple's release from an IVF program after the performance of embryo transfer, GIFT, artificial insemination, or related procedures. An exit interview prepares the couple for their return home and provides valuable feedback to the program.

extracorporeal fertilization   Synonym for IVF.

fallopian tubes   Narrow 4-inch-long structures that lead from either side of the uterus to the ovaries.

falloposcope   A telescopelike instrument that is introduced into the fallopian tubes for diagnostic purposes during falloposcopy.

falloposcopy   A procedure performed at the time of laparoscopy or hysteroscopy, in which a thin telescopelike instrument is introduced into the fallopian tube(s) to evaluate its condition. Falloposcopy even enables the expert reproductive physician to perform surgery inside the fallopian tubes through the falloposcope, thus avoiding the need to open the abdominal cavity except for the small puncture site.

fertility drugs   Natural or synthetic hormones that are administered to a woman to stimulate her ovaries to produce as many mature eggs as possible, or to a man to enhance sperm function or production.

fertilization   The fusion of the sperm and egg to form a zygote (*see also* zygote, conception).

FET   *See* frozen embryo transfer.

fetus   Once the embryo differentiates and begins to take on identifiable humanlike organic form, it is termed a fetus; the fetal stage of development usually begins around the eighth week of pregnancy.

fibroid tumor   A benign tumor in the uterus, which may prevent the embryo from properly implanting into the endometrium or cause pain, bleeding, miscarriage, and symptomatic enlargement of the uterus.

fibrous bands   Scar tissue that may distort the interior of the uterus and prevent the embryo from implanting properly.

fimbriae   Fingerlike protrusions from the ends of the fallopian tubes that retrieve the egg(s) at the time of ovulation.

fluid ultrasonography (FUS)   A simple and relatively painless procedure whereby a sterile solution of saline is injected via a catheter through the cervix and into the uterine cavity. The fluid-distended cavity is examined by vaginal ultrasound. FUS is highly effective in identifying even the smallest intrauterine lesions and can supplant diagnostic hysteroscopy in the preparation of women for IVF.

fluorescence in situ hybridization (FISH)   A chromosome-staining technique that allows for diagnosis of both egg- and sperm-induced embryo chromosomal abnormalities.

follicles   Blisterlike structures within the ovary that contain eggs and that produce female sex hormones.

follicle-stimulating hormone (FSH)   A gonadotropin that is released by the pituitary gland to stimulate the ovaries or testicles. FSH, when marketed in the United States, is also known as Metrodin.

follicular phase insufficiency or defect   An abnormal pattern of estrogen production during the first half of the menstrual cycle, which could result in infertility or recurrent miscarriages.

follicular phase of the menstrual cycle   *See* proliferative phase of the menstrual cycle.

folliculogenesis   The process of follicle growth and development.

fornix (pl. fornices)   Deep recesses in the upper vagina created by the protrusion of the cervix into the roof of the vagina.

frozen embryo transfer (FET)   Process in which previously frozen embryos are thawed and cultured for a few days, and those that attain the blastocyst stage are transferred into the uterus.

FSH   *See* follicle-stimulating hormone.

gamete   The female egg and the male sperm.

gamete intrafallopian transfer (GIFT)   A therapeutic gamete-related technique that involves the injection of one or more eggs mixed with washed, capacitated, and incubated sperm directly into the fallopian tube(s) in the hope that fertilization will occur and that a healthy pregnancy will follow.

gamete micromanipulation   A special procedure performed on eggs to promote IVF in cases where there is severe sperm dysfunction.

gastrulation   The stage of embryonic development in which blastomeres are dedicated to the development of specific organs and structures.

GES   *See* Graduated Embryo Scoring.

gestation   The period from conception to delivery.

gestational surrogacy   The performance of IVF using the prospective parents' gametes and the subsequent transfer of the embryos into the uterus of a third party who thereon would carry the baby to term.

GIFT   *See* gamete intrafallopian transfer.

GnRH   *See* gonadotropin-releasing hormone.

GnRHa   *See* gonadotropin-releasing hormone agonists.

gonadotropin-releasing hormone agonists (GnRHa)   GnRH-like hormones that block the body's release of both FSH and LH. Through blocking LH production, GnRH agonists are capable of improving a woman's response to fertility drugs and may be used in combination with fertility hormones to promote an enhanced response in women who demonstrate resistance to controlled ovarian hyperstimulation. In the United States, GnRH agonists are also known as Lupron, Synarel, and Nafarelin.

gonadotropin-releasing hormone (GnRH)   A "messenger hormone" released by the hypothalamus to influence the production of gonadotropins by the pituitary gland.

gonadotropins   The gonad-stimulating hormones LH and FSH, which are released by the pituitary gland to stimulate the testicles in the man and the ovaries in the woman.

gonads The ovaries and testicles.

gonococcus A bacterium producing gonorrhea, a common venereal disease occurring in both men and women that may cause sterility.

gonorrhea A common venereal disease that may cause sterility in both men and women.

Graduated Embryo Scoring (GES) Method for assessing embryo quality by means of a series of microscopic assessments throughout a period of 72 hours following egg insemination.

growth medium A physiological solution that promotes cleavage and development of the embryo.

Hashimoto's disease An autoimmune disorder.

hatching Opening of the zona (outer shell of the egg) due to expansion of the volume of the embryo through repeated cleavage. It occurs a few days after the embryo arrives or is deposited in the uterus and immediately precedes implantation (*see also* assisted hatching).

hCG *See* human chorionic gonadotropin.

hemi-zona test Used to determine whether sperm are able to attach to or penetrate the surface of human eggs.

heparin A blood-thinning drug that does not cross the placenta and is safe for the baby.

heterotopic pregnancy When implantation occurs in two sites simultaneously (i.e., in the fallopian tube as well as inside the uterine cavity).

high-order multiple pregnancy The presence of three or more gestations within the woman's reproductive tract at the same time.

HLA antigens The imprints of the man's immunologic makeup.

hMG gonadotropins *See* human menopausal gonadotropin.

hormonal insufficiency A condition resulting in infertility and/or miscarriage; in the IVF setting, hormonal insufficiency may be produced by an abnormal response to fertility drugs and may lead to the failure of an embryo to implant because the amount of hormones produced and the timing of their production and release were not perfectly synchronized.

hormone (sex hormone)   Chemicals produced by the testicles, ovaries, and adrenal glands that play a major role in reproduction and sexual identity.

HSG   *See* hysterosalpingogram.

Hühner test   *See* postcoital test.

human chorionic gonadotropin (hCG)   A hormone, produced by the implanting embryo (and subsequently also by the placenta), whose presence in the woman's blood indicates a possible pregnancy; hCG may also be administered to women undergoing stimulation with gonadotropins alone or in combination with other fertility drugs in order to trigger ovulation. Injections of hCG may also be administered to encourage the production of progesterone by the corpus luteum in the hope of promoting implantation following embryo transfer and thereby reducing the incidence of spontaneous miscarriage in a pregnancy resulting from IVF. In such situations, the hormone hCG is derived from the urine of pregnant women.

human menopausal gonadotropin (hMG)   A natural hormone that is administered either alone or in combination with other fertility drugs to induce ovulation of more than one egg. The hormone hMG is derived from the urine of menopausal women.

hydrosalpinx   A condition in which the fallopian tubes are distended with fluid.

hypothalamus   A small area in the midportion of the brain that, together with the pituitary gland, regulates the formation and release of many hormones in the body, including estrogen and progesterone by the ovaries and testosterone by the testes.

hysterosalpingogram (HSG)   A procedure used to assess the shape of the uterine cavity and the patency of the fallopian tubes; it involves injecting a dye into the uterus via the vagina and cervix, and tracking the dye's pathway by a series of X-rays.

hysteroscope   A lighted, telescopelike instrument that is passed through the cervix into the uterus, enabling the surgeon to examine the cervical canal and the inside of the uterus for defects or disease.

hysteroscopy   Examination of the cervical canal and inside of the uterus for defects, by means of the hysteroscope. Surgery designed to correct such defects can be performed through the hysteroscope during this procedure, thereby often making more invasive abdominal surgery unnecessary.

ICSI *See* intracytoplasmic sperm injection.

immature oocyte (or egg) retrieval The retrieval of numerous healthy but immature eggs from women who had not received any fertility drugs in advance of the egg retrieval; these eggs are subjected to a complex process of maturation in the laboratory and are then fertilized using ICSI.

immunologic implant failure Failure of the embryo to attach properly to the uterine wall, in the presence of antithyroid antibodies (ATA).

implantation The process that occurs when the embryo burrows into the endometrium and eventually connects to the mother's circulatory system.

inclusive pregnancy rates Pregnancy success reports that combine rates for both clinical and chemical pregnancies and do not distinguish between the two.

infertility The inability to conceive after one full year of normal, regular heterosexual intercourse without the use of contraception.

inner cell mass (ICM) The specialized cells on the inner surface of the morula that eventually develop into the fetus.

insemination In the laboratory, the addition of a drop or two of the medium containing capacitated sperm to a petri dish containing the egg in order to achieve fertilization. Also refers to placement of sperm into the woman's reproductive tract.

insemination medium A liquid that bathes and nourishes the eggs and embryos in the petri dish just as the mother's body fluids sustain them in nature.

intracytoplasmic sperm injection (ICSI) A form of micromanipulation whereby a single sperm is captured in a thin glass needle and injected directly into the ooplasm of the egg. Usually used to assist fertilization in couples suffering from severe sperm dysfunction.

intrauterine insemination (IUI) The injection of sperm, processed in the laboratory, into the uterus by means of a catheter directed through the cervix; enables sperm to reach and fertilize the egg more easily or to bypass hostile cervical mucus.

intravaginal insemination (IVI)   The injection of semen (usually donor semen) into the vagina in direct proximity to the cervix in the hope that pregnancy will occur.

intravenous immunoglobin (IVIG)   A sterile protein preparation derived from human blood that may offset or counter the anti-implantation effects associated with reproductive immunologic deficiencies.

invasive procedure   Any operative procedure, major or minor, that traverses body tissues. In the case of fertility-related treatments, a surgical procedure that requires that one or more punctures or incisions be made in the woman's abdomen.

in vitro fertilization (IVF or IVF/ET)   Literally "fertilization in glass," IVF is comprised of several basic steps: the woman is given fertility drugs that stimulate her ovaries to produce a number of mature eggs; at the proper time, the eggs are retrieved by suction through a needle that has been inserted into her ovaries; the eggs are fertilized in a petri dish, or in a test tube, in the laboratory with her partner's or donor sperm; and subsequently the embryos are transferred into the body.

in vivo fertilization   Fertilization inside the body.

isohormones   Similarly structured components that have different levels of biological activity; the influence of isohormones may be responsible for the variations in potency among different batches of gonadotropins such as hMG and purified FSH.

IUI   *See* intrauterine insemination.

IVF third-party parenting   A situation in which an individual other than one of the aspiring parents provides gametes (as with sperm or ovum donation) or a uterus, and the woman who will carry the baby to term undergoes embryo transfer.

IVF or IVF/ET   *See* in vitro fertilization.

IVF surrogacy   Synonym for gestational surrogacy.

IVI   *See* intravaginal insemination.

IVIG   *See* intravenous immunoglobin.

labia majora   The hair-covered outer lips of the external portion of the female reproductive tract.

labia minora   The small inner lips of the outer female reproductive tract, partially hidden by the labia majora.

laparoscope A long, thin telescopelike instrument containing a high-intensity light source and a system of lenses that enables the surgeon to examine the abdominal/pelvic cavity and to perform other diagnostic or surgical procedures under direct vision without necessitating major surgery.

laparoscopy A surgical procedure using the laparoscope. Laparoscopy may be used for egg retrieval, diagnostic evaluation, reparative surgery, and various other fertility procedures. Because of its dual abilities to enable the physician to assess tubal patency and visualize the abdominal cavity, laparoscopy has largely replaced hysterosalpingography as the most popular method of assessing the anatomical integrity of the reproductive tract (*See also* augmented laparoscopy). Once the favored procedure for egg retrieval, laparoscopic egg retrieval has been supplanted by ultrasound-guided needle-aspiration egg retrieval.

laparotomy A procedure in which an incision is made in the abdomen to expose the abdominal contents for diagnosis or surgery.

Letrozole An oral ovulation-induction agent that inhibits aromatase, an enzyme that promotes estrogen production by the ovaries. This causes a rebound release of FSH and LH that promotes follicle growth followed by ovulation.

LH *See* luteinizing hormone.

lithotomy Position that a woman is asked to assume in order to undergo a gynecological examination or other procedure, such as embryo transfer or vaginal ultrasound examination.

LUFS *See* luteinized unruptured follicle syndrome.

luteal-phase insufficiency or defect The inadequate production of hormones during the second phase of the menstrual cycle, which may result in infertility or miscarriage.

luteal phase of the menstrual cycle *See* secretory phase of the menstrual cycle.

luteinized unruptured follicle syndrome (LUFS) When hormonal changes associated with ovulation and a commensurate rise in the blood progesterone level take place but the egg is not released from the ovary. Also known as "trapped ovulation."

luteinizing hormone (LH) A gonadotropin released by the pituitary gland to stimulate the ovaries and testicles.

macrophages   Cells of the immune system that destroy invading organisms or foreign proteins.

male subfertility   Less than optimal sperm quality, including configuration, motility, and count (number produced in a semen specimen), that reduces the chance of conception without completely preventing its spontaneous occurrence.

meiosis   The process of reducing and dividing the chromosomes in both the sperm and egg, which occurs immediately prior to and during fertilization.

menarche   The onset of a woman's menstruation.

menopause   The period of a woman's life that begins with the total cessation of menstruation, usually between the ages of 40 and 55.

menstrual cycle   The time that elapses between menstrual periods. The average cycle is 28 days, with ovulation usually occurring at the midpoint (around the 14th day).

menstruation   The monthly flow of blood when pregnancy does not occur; the flow is comprised of about two-thirds of the endometrium and blood, often including the unfertilized egg or unimplanted embryo.

MESA   *See* microsurgical epididymal aspiration.

messenger hormones   *See* gonadotropin-releasing hormones (GnRH).

micromanipulation   A term used to describe a variety of mechanical procedures used to promote the entry of sperm into the egg. Also called assisted fertilization.

microorganelles   Tiny intracellular factories that provide energy and perform metabolic functions in the egg, where the microorganelles are located largely in the ooplasm.

microsurgical epididymal aspiration (MESA)   A procedure that involves aspirating sperm from sperm-collecting ducts on the surface of the testicles.

miscarriage   Spontaneous expulsion of the products of conception from the uterus in the first half of pregnancy.

mitosis   The identical replication of cells by cleavage; mitosis is the process responsible for the growth and development of all tissues.

mock embryo transfer   A trial procedure wherein a thin catheter is introduced via the cervix into the uterine cavity. It is intended to simulate embryo transfer and evaluate the potential for embryo transfer.

morphology (of sperm) The percentage of sperm that have a normal vs. abnormal shape, structure, or configuration.

morula An early phase during which the developing embryo, which contains a large number of blastomeres, resembles a mulberry.

motility The ability of sperm to move and progress forward through the reproductive tract and fertilize the egg; sperm motility can be assessed microscopically.

multiple pregnancy The presence of more than one gestation within the woman's reproductive tract at the same time.

myceles Microfibers within the cervical mucus that sperm must swim through to reach the uterus; the woman's hormonal environment determines whether the arrangement of the myceles will facilitate or inhibit passage of the sperm. Around the time of ovulation the myceles are arranged in a parallel fashion so that sperm can swim between them in order to reach the uterus; it is believed that capacitation is promoted during that process.

natural cycle IVF A situation in which one or two eggs are harvested from a woman's ovaries during the natural menstrual cycle and are then subjected to IVF and embryo transfer. Success rates are much lower than with conventional IVF.

nonpigmented endometriosis A condition in which endometriotic deposits in the pelvis cannot be seen at the time of laparoscopy or laparotomy because blood pigment has not been deposited in these lesions. The condition is believed to often precede the development of visible lesions.

nucleus Structure in the cell that bears the chromosomes.

oocyte *See* egg.

ooplasm Nurturing material around the nucleus of the egg that contains micoorganelles and nurtures the zygote and embryo after fertilization.

operative laparoscope A laparoscope that has been modified to allow passage of a double-bored needle or surgical instruments through a groove or sleeve adjacent to the instrument (*see also* laparoscope).

organic pelvic disease The presence of structural damage in the pelvis due to trauma, inflammation, tumors, congenital defects, or degenerative disease.

Outcome-Based Reimbursement (OBR) A financial plan whereby full payment for IVF is only made in the event of a baby being born following the transfer of all embryos (over one or more months of treatment).

ovarian stroma The ovarian tissue surrounding the follicles that produces hormones.

ovaries Two white, almond-sized structures, the female counterpart of the testicles, that are attached to each side of the pelvis adjacent to the ends of the fallopian tubes; the ovaries both release eggs and discharge sex hormones into the bloodstream.

ovulation The process by which an ovary releases one or more eggs.

ovum *See* egg.

partial zona dissection A mechanical form of assisted hatching in which part of the zona (outer shell of the egg) is dissected away in order to promote hatching.

patency Openness, freedom from blockage (particularly referring to the fallopian tubes).

PCR *See* polymerase chain reaction.

PCT test *See* postcoital test.

peeling Removal of the corona radiata from the embryo by flushing the embryo through a syringe or pipette, or by microdissection using fine instruments. An embryo often must first be peeled before it is possible to determine whether fertilization and cleavage have occurred.

pelvic inflammatory disease (PID) Results from infection of pelvic structures, especially the fallopian tubes, and which can inhibit the passage of eggs, sperm, and embryos in a timely manner to and from the uterine cavity, thus compromising fertility.

penis The male external sex organ.

Percoll A chemical substance through which sperm are passed to enhance fertilization potential.

perineum The outer portion of the fibromuscular wall and skin that separate the anus and rectum from the vagina and vulva.

peristaltic movements of fallopian tubes Mechanism by which the fallopian tubes contract in a purposeful and rhythmical way to transport sperm, eggs, and embryos in a timely manner so as to promote fertilization and, ultimately, implantation.

peritoneal cavity The abdominal cavity that contains pelvic organs, bowel, stomach, liver, kidneys, adrenal glands, spleen, etc., and is lined by a membrane called the peritoneum.

perivitelline membrane Membrane that separates the ooplasm and nuclear material from the zona pellucida in the human egg.

phrenic nerve Nerve that may be irritated by trapped gas or blood during laparoscopy or following internal bleeding, resulting in subsequent pain in the shoulder, arm, and neck (most commonly on the right side).

PID *See* pelvic inflammatory disease.

pituitary gland A small, grapelike structure hanging from the base of the brain that, together with the hypothalamus, produces and regulates the release of many hormones in the body.

placenta The uterine factory that nourishes the fetus throughout pregnancy and is connected to the baby's navel via the umbilical cord.

placentation Formation and attachment of the placenta to the uterine wall.

plasma membrane Double-layered membrane that envelops the entire sperm.

polar body biopsy Biopsy of egg-derived chromosome populations within 36 hours of fertilization for the diagnosis of both egg- and sperm-induced embryo aneuploidies.

polycystic ovarian disease (PCOS) Condition in which the ovaries develop multiple small cysts; it is often associated with abnormal or absent ovulation and, accordingly, with infertility.

polymerase chain reaction (PCR) Technology involving identification and amplification of one or more gene loci on the chromosome.

polyploidy Situation in which more than two pronuclei (conglomerates of chromosomal material) are present; because of this, the zygote will not produce a viable embryo.

polyps (uterine) Outgrowths that protrude into the uterus and may cause pain and bleeding or prevent an embryo from implanting.

postcoital test (PCT)   Assessment of the cervical mucus after intercourse to evaluate the quality of the mucus and mucus-sperm interaction; also known as the Hühner test.

pregnancy-specific glycoprotein (SP-1)   A hormone that appears in the blood only a few days later than hCG during pregnancy. May be measured instead of hCG to diagnose pregnancy.

pre-implantation genetic diagnosis (PGD)   A new diagnostic technology involving chromosome and genetic assessment of the embryo in order to determine its health and potential to develop into a healthy offspring. A procedure currently used to determine the sex of the embryo and to diagnose a variety of genetic disorders.

progesterone   A primary female sex hormone produced by the corpus luteum that induces secretory changes in the glands of the endometrium. Progesterone may also be given by injection or in the form of vaginal suppositories to enhance implantation and reduce the risk of miscarriage.

prolactin   A hormone produced by the brain that may influence the activity of FSH on the ovaries.

proliferative phase of the menstrual cycle   Usually, the first half of the menstrual cycle, when the endometrium grows under the influence of estrogen and the follicles develop; also known as the follicular phase.

prolonged coasting   The discontinuation of gonadotropin medication and deferring hCG administration for a number of days, while continuing GnRH agonist therapy in cases where severe ovarian hyperstimulation occurs following COH in preparation for IVF.

prostaglandins   Natural hormones contained in a multitude of cells in the body as well as in the seminal fluid. The placement of semen, which contains seminal fluid with prostaglandins, directly in the uterus in quantities greater than 0.2 ml can cause life-threatening shock.

prostate gland   Gland in the male reproductive tract that secretes a milky substance that nurtures and promotes survival of sperm. The combination of sperm and milky fluid that is ejaculated during erotic experiences is known as semen.

purified FSH   A fertility hormone derived by processing and purifying gonadotropins to eliminate the LH component.

quantitative beta hCG blood pregnancy test Test that detects and measures the amount of hCG (produced by an implanting embryo) in the woman's blood. Measured about 11 and 13 days after embryo transfer, it can diagnose a possible pregnancy before the woman has missed a menstrual period.

rectum Lower portion of the large intestine that connects to the anal canal.

reproductive cloning Replication of an existing animal by swapping its DNA with the DNA in an egg from the same species; the resulting embryo is either transferred directly to the uterus or allowed to divide several times before being transferred; sheep and other mammals have been cloned with this procedure.

Resolve, Inc. One of the largest and most reputable fertility support groups in the United States; its national office is in Somerville, Mass.

retrograde ejaculation A condition, sometimes caused by a spinal cord injury or following removal of a diseased prostate gland, in which the man ejaculates backward into the bladder rather than outward through the penis. It may cause infertility but can be treated by inseminating the woman with sperm separated from urine the man would pass immediately following orgasm.

salpingoscopy A procedure involving the introduction of a thin fiber-optic instrument into the fallopian tube or tubes to promote visualization of the tubal lining. It is usually performed during laparoscopy but may also be performed through a hysteroscope.

salpingostomy A form of tubal surgery in which the end of the fallopian tube(s) is opened at the time of laparoscopy or laparotomy, using small surgical stitches or a laser.

SART *See* Society of Assisted Reproductive Technology.

sclerotherapy for ovarian endometriomas Needle aspiration of the liquid content of the endometriotic cyst, followed by the injection of 5 percent solution of tetracycline into the cyst cavity.

scrotum Pouch in which the male's testicles are suspended outside the body.

secretory phase of the menstrual cycle The second half of the menstrual cycle, which begins after ovulation under the influence of estrogen and progesterone produced by the corpus luteum; the term *secretory* is derived from the secretion by the endometrium of nutrients that will sustain an embryo; also known as the luteal phase.

selective reduction of pregnancy   Prior to completion of the third month of pregnancy, reduction of the number of fetuses in a large multiple pregnancy by injecting a chemical substance under ultrasound guidance; the fetus or fetuses succumb almost immediately and are absorbed by the body. It may be considered a life-saving measure for the remaining fetuses in high-multiple pregnancies (triplets and greater) and reduces the risk to the mother.

semen   The combination of sperm, seminal fluid, and other male reproductive secretions.

seminal fluid   Milky fluid produced by the seminal vesicles that is ejaculated during erotic experiences (*see also* semen).

seminal vesicles   Glands in the male reproductive tract that secrete a milky substance that nurtures and promotes survival of sperm.

sHLA-G   *See* soluble human leukocyte antigen-G.

Society for Assisted Reproductive Technology (SART)   Affiliated with the American Society for Reproductive Medicine, SART provides information about IVF programs and compiles a registry of audited IVF results from participating programs.

soluble human leukocyte antigen-G   A genetic marker excreted into the growth medium of the petri dish and measured to identify those embryos most likely to produce a pregnancy.

sonohysterogram   *See* fluid ultrasonography.

sperm   The male gamete; spermatozoa.

sperm antibody test   Test that determines whether either partner's blood or the woman's cervical mucus contains antibodies to sperm.

sperm count   A basic fertility-assessment test of sperm function, primarily involving counting the number of sperm, assessing their motility and progression, and evaluating their overall structure and form.

spontaneous menstrual abortion   An early miscarriage occurring at the time of menstruation without the woman's menstrual period being delayed.

SP-I   *See* pregnancy-specific glycoprotein.

sterility   *See* infertility.

stimulation   Induction of the development of a number of follicles in response to the administration of fertility drugs (*see also* controlled ovarian hyperstimulation and superovulation).

subzonal insertion (SUZI)   The direct injection of one or more sperm into the perivitelline space to promote fertilization. It is a form of micromanipulation.

superovulation   The ovulation of more than one egg induced through the administration of fertility drugs (*see also* controlled ovarian hyperstimulation and stimulation).

surrogacy   Situation in which an infertile woman uses someone else's uterus to carry a child to term. Surrogacy can be divided into (1) cases in which the surrogate mother contributes biologically to the offspring by providing her own eggs (classic surrogacy) and (2) cases in which the surrogate does not contribute biologically and therefore must undergo IVF (gestational surrogacy).

SUZI   *See* subzonal insertion.

syphilis   A life-endangering venereal disease that in its late stages attacks most systems in the body, including the cardiovascular and central nervous systems.

testes   *See* testicles.

testicles   The male counterparts of the female ovaries; located in the scrotum, the testicles produce sperm and male hormones such as testosterone.

testicular sperm aspiration (TESA)   A procedure performed on an outpatient basis (usually under local anesthesia) where sperm are aspirated from the sperm duct for use in ICSI.

testicular sperm extraction (TESE)   A procedure performed on an outpatient basis (usually under local anesthesia) where one or more hair-thin biopsy specimens are removed and delivered to the embryology laboratory for sperm to be removed for ICSI.

testosterone   The predominant male sex hormone, which influences the production and maturation of sperm.

test yolk buffer   A sperm-enhancement solution derived from the yolk of a chicken egg.

therapeutic gamete-related technologies   Procedures involving the use of gametes to enhance the chance of conception through subsequent insemination, or transfer of eggs and/or sperm into the woman's uterus, fallopian tubes, or peritoneal cavity.

therapeutic hysteroscopy A procedure, usually performed under general anesthesia, in which a clear liquid is injected into the uterine cavity via the hysteroscope. This permits exposure of surface lesions inside the uterus or cervix via X-ray. These lesions can be treated surgically through excision, obliteration, transection, etc.

third-party parenting Any situation in which an individual other than the aspiring parents assists by providing gametes (as with sperm and ovum donation) or a uterus in order to help the couple have a baby.

thrombophilia The inherited tendency to develop blood clots too easily.

thyroid-stimulating hormone (TSH) A hormone produced by the pituitary gland that stimulates the release of thyroid hormone by the thyroid gland.

TPI *See* transperitoneal insemination.

transabdominal egg retrieval An ultrasound-guided egg-retrieval procedure in which the needle is passed through the abdominal wall and a full bladder into the ovarian follicles; it has largely been supplanted by transvaginal egg retrieval.

transcervical Refers to the physiological or surgical pathway whereby secretions, organisms, sperm, or surgical instrumentation passes from the vagina into the uterus.

transmyometrial embryo transfer A procedure that transfers embryos to the uterus via a needle and/or catheter introduced through the uterine wall (myometrium) rather than through the cervix. It is used in situations where severe narrowing of the cervix negates the performance of conventional embryo transfer.

transperitoneal insemination (TPI) The injection of washed sperm through a syringe into the woman's pelvic cavity at the time of expected ovulation to promote conception; it may be combined with intrauterine insemination.

transurethral egg retrieval An ultrasound-guided egg retrieval procedure in which the needle is passed through the urethra and the bladder wall into the ovaries; it has largely been supplanted by transvaginal egg retrieval.

transvaginal egg retrieval An ultrasound-guided egg retrieval procedure in which a needle is passed through the back or side of the woman's vagina into her ovaries. It is the most commonly performed egg retrieval procedure today.

trapped ovulation *See* Luteinized Unruptured Follicle Syndrome.

treatment cycle The menstrual cycle during which a particular fertility treatment, such as IVF, IUI, AID, GIFT, etc., was performed.

trophoblast The root system of the conceptus, which subsequently develops into the placenta.

tubal abortion A pregnancy that gained early attachment to a fallopian tube's inner lining is absorbed before the woman even knows that she is pregnant.

tubal embryo transfer (TET) A procedure, usually performed via laparoscopy, in which one or more embryos are inserted in the fallopian tube(s) via a thin catheter a few days following egg retrieval; also known as zygote intrafallopian transfer (ZIFT).

tubal pregnancy *See* ectopic pregnancy.

tubal reanastomosis A surgical procedure in which the fallopian tubes are reconnected, reestablishing patency. Usually performed after a previous tubal ligation (sterilization).

tuboscopy A procedure in which a thin fiber-optic telescope is passed into the fallopian tube(s) to evaluate their inner structure.

UCFD *See* ultrasound color flow Doppler.

ultrasound A painless diagnostic procedure that transforms high-frequency sound waves as they travel through body tissue and fluid into images on a TV-like screen; it enables the physician to clearly identify structures within the body and to guide instruments during certain procedures. Ultrasound is also used to diagnose a clinical pregnancy.

ultrasound color flow Doppler (UCFD) A means of measuring uterine blood flow.

unexplained infertility Infertility whose cause cannot be readily determined by conventional diagnostic procedures; this occurs in about 10 percent of all infertile couples.

ureaplasma A microorganism that occurs in the reproductive tracts of males and females; it may interfere with sperm transport and/or embryo implantation. It might also be responsible for early miscarriages.

urethra   The canal-like structure through which urine passes from the bladder and through which semen passes during ejaculation.

urine ovulation test   A simple test that can pinpoint the time of presumed ovulation; frequent charting of the test results detects the surge of LH that triggers ovulation.

uterus   A muscular organ that enlarges during pregnancy from its normal pearlike shape and size to accommodate a full-term pregnancy.

vagina   The narrow passage that leads from the vulva to the cervix. The vagina's elastic tissue, muscle, and skin have enormous ability to stretch so as to accommodate the penis during the sex act and the passage of a baby during childbirth.

varicocele   A collection of dilated veins around the testicles that hinders sperm function, possibly through increasing the temperature in the scrotum.

vas deferens   Tube that connects the epididymis with the urethra in the male reproductive tract.

vasectomy   Surgery to block the male's sperm ducts for the purpose of birth control.

vestibule   The cleft between the labia minora; the entrance to the vagina.

vulva   The external portion of the female reproductive tract.

warfarin   A blood-thinning drug.

washing (sperm washing)   The processing of a semen specimen in a centrifuge in order to separate the sperm from the semen specimen.

yellow body   *See* corpus luteum.

ZIFT   *See* zygote intrafallopian transfer.

zona-cumulus complex   The mass of cells (zona pellucida and cumulus mass) through which the sperm must pass to reach the egg.

zona drilling   A form of micromanipulation whereby a small hole is made in the zona pellucida to promote free entry of a sperm into the egg.

zygote intrafallopian transfer (ZIFT)   Another name for tubal embryo transfer.

INDEX

Italic page numbers indicate illustrations or captions.
Boldface page numbers indicate glossary terms.

G

H

I

K

L